Essential Examination

OTHER BOOKS FROM SCION

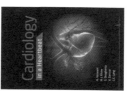

9781907904257

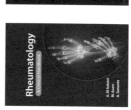

9781907904035

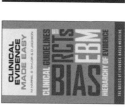

9781907904202

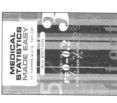

9781907904264

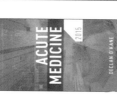

9781907904783

3rd Edition

Essential Examination

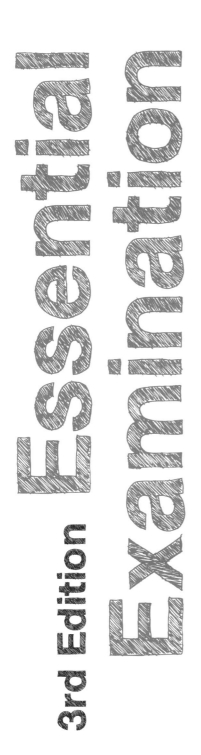

Alasdair K. B. Ruthven MBChB (Hons) BSc (Hons)

Specialist Trainee in Anaesthetics, Royal Infirmary of Edinburgh, UK

Step-by-step guides to clinical examination scenarios
with practical tips and key facts for OSCEs

Scion

© **Scion Publishing Ltd, 2016**

Third Edition published in 2016
Second Edition published in 2010; reprinted 2011, 2012, 2013, 2014, 2015
First Edition published in 2009 by Alasdair Ruthven

ISBN 978 1 907904 10 3

A CIP catalogue record for this book is available from the British Library.

Scion Publishing Limited

The Old Hayloft, Vantage Business Park, Bloxham Road, Banbury, Oxfordshire OX16 9UX

www.scionpublishing.com

Important Note from the Publisher

The information contained within this book was obtained by Scion Publishing Limited from sources believed by us to be reliable. However, while every effort has been made to ensure its accuracy, no responsibility for loss or injury whatsoever occasioned to any person acting or refraining from action as a result of information contained herein can be accepted by the author or publishers.

Readers should remember that medicine is a constantly evolving science and while the author and publishers have ensured that all dosages, applications and practices are based on current indications, there may be specific practices which differ between communities. You should always follow the guidelines laid down by the manufacturers of specific products and the relevant authorities in the country in which you are practising.

Although every effort has been made to ensure that all owners of copyright material have been acknowledged in this publication, we would be pleased to acknowledge in subsequent reprints or editions any omissions brought to our attention.

Typeset by Phoenix Photosetting, Chatham, Kent, UK

Printed in the UK

CONTENTS

PREFACE

BACKGROUND

Essential Examination began life as a set of notes I produced for my undergraduate exams. At that time I was unable to find a book that succinctly laid out the full sequence for examination of one body system on one page. This format remains the key feature of the book, which has steadily expanded over the past 10 years. Although the content has been extensively reviewed, refined and updated, much of it is still presented in ways that helped me to remember it at medical school.

WHAT'S NOT INCLUDED

To use this book requires a good baseline understanding of the physiology and pathophysiology of the systems considered. Some detail has been omitted intentionally – for example, nowhere is the exact method of examining for flapping tremor explained. It is assumed that core skills like this become second nature as they are taught time and time again in clinical teaching. This makes space for other useful information, and detailed descriptions of less familiar elements of examination where the margins between looking slick and looking awkward are narrower. Often there are many ways of examining for the same thing in medicine; in such cases I have described either the method preferred by specialists, or where no consensus exists, the method that I find the easiest.

APPEARANCE & CONDUCT

It goes without saying that when examining patients, in an OSCE or not, you should appear smart (this includes hair, facial hair and clothing) and be 'bare below the elbows'. Always be polite and courteous, and ensure you do not cause any harm, e.g. before palpating an abdomen or manoeuvring a joint, ask if it has been painful. Respect your patients' dignity and avoid unnecessary exposure; where necessary for a thorough examination, minimize the duration of exposure and always ensure privacy. A chaperone should be present for all intimate examinations, and you may consider using one in other scenarios (e.g. a male clinician examining a young female's abdomen). In an OSCE, have a very low threshold to mention that you would consider having a chaperone.

OSCE TIPS

Often in an OSCE you will not be asked to complete the full examination of a particular body system. Instead, you may be asked to complete part of that examination (e.g. rather than 'examine the cardiovascular system', simply 'examine the precordium'). However, in order to do this you must draw from a baseline knowledge of the examination in its entirety. Alternatively you may be asked to examine multiple systems at once (e.g. a cardio-respiratory examination). *Always* listen to what the examiner asks, and clarify if necessary. Make sure you have practised these types of scenarios.

Usually you should examine from the patient's right-hand side, although some examinations require you to move around the bed. Remember that many examinations follow a standard sequence, for example:

Core medical: peripheral signs – inspection – palpation – percussion – auscultation
Neurological: inspection – tone – power – reflexes – sensation – co-ordination
Musculoskeletal: look – feel – move – special tests – function – check distal neurovascular integrity

If you get lost in an examination (so easy to do under the pressure of assessment), default to these basic frameworks to get yourself back on track. Some examinations, of course, follow their own unique sequence; these are the most difficult to learn and so you must become very familiar with them.

At the end of your examination, present your findings clearly and succinctly. Always have some concluding remarks up your sleeve too – it's a good way to finish off, and gives the impression that you really know your stuff.

Finally, remember that in order to pass you do not need to recall every single piece of information contained in this book – a slick, comprehensive clinical examination combined with some solid core knowledge is certainly enough. The old saying that difficult questions mean you are doing well is very true – don't forget it!

Good luck!

A.K.B. Ruthven
October 2015

If you have any questions or comments regarding the book, please email me at: author@essentialexamination.com

ACKNOWLEDGEMENTS

I would like to thank my many clinical tutors and colleagues for their role in the creation and development of this book. Thanks in particular to the following people for their help and suggestions:

Mr Mark Gaston   Musculoskeletal
Mr Zahid Raza   Circulation
Dr Ingibjorg Gudmundsdottir   Cardiovascular
Dr Kirsty Dundas   Pregnant abdomen
Dr Aoife Casey   Neonatal

I would also like to thank Mr Andrew Ker and Dr Angela Waugh for modelling in the musculoskeletal examination photos.

Finally, I would like to express my appreciation for all the undergraduates who have supported the project with their recommendations and abundant enthusiasm.

FOREWORD

The most important core skills for medical students to master are history taking and clinical examination. This conveniently ring-bound text has been written with the philosophy that clinical skills can be more effectively honed at the bedside, and as such it should be used as a constant companion on the ward and in the consulting room.

Each section of the book covers the physical examination of a body system, beginning with a detailed step-by-step description of the examination method, complemented by practical tips and key facts. Detailed information relating to that examination is provided in the form of helpful illustrations, diagrams and tables with space for you to add your own notes.

This book is intended primarily to be used by medical students in their 'clinical' years who, having attained a sound grasp of clinical science and disease processes are beginning to hone examination techniques. It is of particular use to those who are preparing for final assessments and practising techniques during revision.

Professor Mike Ford
Edinburgh, 2010

ABBREVIATIONS

ΔΔ	Differential diagnosis
#	Fracture
♂	Male
♀	Female
[pxx]	See page xx
2°	Secondary to
Ca	Cancer
Pt	Patient
Rx	Treatment
[⊃]	See over: check in Notes
AAA	Abdominal aortic aneurysm
ABG	Arterial blood gas
ABPI	Ankle brachial pressure index
AC	Acromio-clavicular (joint)
ACEi	ACE inhibitor
ACL	Anterior cruciate ligament (of knee)
ACS	Acute coronary syndrome
ACTH	Adrenocorticotrophic hormone
AF	Atrial fibrillation
AKI	Acute kidney injury
ALS	Advanced life support
A–P	Anterior–posterior (diameter)
APKD	Adult polycystic kidney disease
AR	Aortic regurgitation
AS	Aortic stenosis
ASIS	Anterior superior iliac spine
AV	Arterio-venous (malformation / fistula)
AVN	Avascular necrosis
BLS	Basic life support
BP	Blood pressure
CABG	Coronary artery bypass graft
CCF	Congestive cardiac failure
CFA	Cryptogenic fibrosing alveolitis
CHD	Congenital heart disease
CKD	Chronic kidney disease
CLD	Chronic liver disease
CML	Chronic myeloid leukaemia
CN	Cranial nerve
CNS	Central nervous system
COPD	Chronic obstructive pulmonary disease
CRF	Chronic renal failure
CRP	C-reactive protein
LLETZ	Large loop excision of the transformation zone
LLSE	Lower left sternal edge
LMN	Lower motor neurone
LMWH	Low molecular weight heparin
LSV	Long saphenous vein
LV	Left ventricle
LVH	Left ventricular hypertrophy
MCL	Medial collateral ligament (of knee)
MI	Myocardial infarction
MND	Motor neurone disease
MNG	Multinodular goitre
MR	Mitral regurgitation
MRA	Magnetic resonance angiography
MRI	Magnetic resonance imaging (scan)
MS	Mitral stenosis / Multiple sclerosis
NOF	Neck of femur (fracture)
NSAID	Non-steroidal anti-inflammatory drug
OA	Osteoarthritis
OCP	Oral contraceptive pill
PBC	Primary biliary cirrhosis
PCA	Posterior communicating artery
PCI	Percutaneous coronary intervention
PCL	Posterior cruciate ligament (of knee)
PDA	Patent ductus arteriosus
PE	Pulmonary embolism
PEFR	Peak expiratory flow rate
PFTs	Pulmonary function tests
PIPJ	Proximal interphalangeal joint
PND	Paroxysmal nocturnal dyspnoea
PNS	Peripheral nervous system
PR	Pulmonary regurgitation / Per-rectal (examination)
PSC	Primary sclerosing cholangitis

CRT	Capillary refill time
CSF	Cerebrospinal fluid
CT	Computerised tomography (scan)
CVS	Cardiovascular system
CXR	Chest X-ray
DDH	Developmental dislocation of the hip
DHS	Dynamic hip screw
DIPJ	Distal interphalangeal joint
DM	Diabetes mellitus
DMARD	Disease-modifying anti-rheumatic drug
DMD	Duchenne muscular dystrophy
DVT	Deep vein thrombosis
EAA	Extrinsic allergic alveolitis
EBV	Epstein–Barr virus
ECG	Electrocardiogram
ESR	Erythrocyte sedimentation rate
FAP	Familial adenomatous polyposis
FNA	Fine needle aspiration
GCA	Giant cell arteritis
GFR	Glomerular filtration rate
GH	Growth hormone
GI	Gastrointestinal
GTN	Glyceryl trinitrate (spray)
Hb	Haemoglobin
HB	Heart block
HCC	Hepatocellular carcinoma
HDU	High dependency unit
HOCM	Hypertrophic obstructive cardiomyopathy
HS	Heart sound
HTN	Hypertension
IBD	Inflammatory bowel disease
ICD	Implantable cardioverter-defibrillator
ICU	Intensive care unit
IE	Infective endocarditis
ILD	Interstitial lung disease
IM	Intramuscular
INO	Intranuclear ophthalmoplegia
IVDU	Intravenous drug user
JVP	Jugular venous pulse
LCL	Lateral collateral ligament (of knee)
LHF	Left heart failure
LHS	Left-hand side
LIF	Left iliac fossa
LIMA	Left internal mammary artery
PVD	Peripheral vascular disease
RR	Respiratory rate
R-R	Radio-radial (delay)
RA	Rheumatoid arthritis
RAAS	Renin–angiotensin–aldosterone system
RAPD	Relative afferent papillary defect
RHF	Right heart failure
RIF	Right iliac fossa
ROM	Range of motion
RTA	Road traffic accident
RUQ	Right upper quadrant
RVH	Right ventricular hypertrophy
SBP	Spontaneous bacterial peritonitis
SC	Subcutaneous
SCDC	Subacute combined degeneration of the cord
SCLC	Small-cell lung cancer
SCM	Sternocleidomastoid
SE	Side-effects
SLE	Systemic lupus erythematosus
SOB	Shortness of breath
SFJ	Sapheno-femoral junction
SPJ	Sapheno-popliteal junction
SpO_2	Peripheral oxygen saturation
SSV	Short saphenous vein
SUFE	Slipped upper femoral epiphysis
SVC	Superior vena cava
TAH	Total abdominal hysterectomy
TAVI	Transcatheter aortic valve implantation
TB	Tuberculosis
TFTs	Thyroid function tests
TIPSS	Transjugular intrahepatic porto-systemic shunt
TR	Tricuspid regurgitation
TS	Tricuspid stenosis
TSH	Thyroid stimulating hormone
U+Es	Urea and electrolytes
UC	Ulcerative colitis
UMN	Upper motor neurone
USS	Ultrasound scan
VEB	Ventricular ectopic beat
VR	Vocal resonance
VSD	Ventricular septal defect
VT	Ventricular tachycardia
WCC	White cell count

HOW TO USE THE BOOK

Each section contains a clear, step-by-step guide to that particular examination, including useful things to say to the patient (or an examiner), detailed descriptions of special tests, etc. In the right-hand column is a collection of key information: potential findings, differential diagnoses of clinical signs and practical tips. On the following pages is a series of facts relating to that particular examination, selected because of the regularity with which they are asked about in bedside teaching and OSCEs. In some sections there are also tips on how to present your findings succinctly – a skill which is crucial to master for exam success.

To get the most out of *Essential Examination* first familiarise yourself with the examinations and learn some of the associated facts. The key is then *practice*. Spend as much time as you can with your clinical tutors and fellow students examining patients (and each other), and quizzing one another on the information in the right-hand columns and on the notes for each section. After every examination, practice presenting your findings too.

Space is included to add your own notes, and I would highly recommend doing so. Anything that helps your understanding or ability to recall information will really be of benefit to you during an OSCE.

	Action / Examine for	ΔΔ / Potential findings / Extra information
Introduction	• Wash / gel hands • Introduce yourself, confirm pt, explain examination & gain consent • Expose & position pt (top off, supine at 45°)	→ Consider chaperone → Bra should be removed once you get to precordium in ♀
End of the bed	• General appearance – well / unwell / distressed / in pain • Oxygen, fluids & medications, *walking aids, ECG monitors* ☞	→ *Marfan's / Down's – congenital cardiac problem* → GTN spray → *check of majatic valves.*
Hands	• Feel temperature & check capillary refill time • Peripheral cyanosis • Tendon xanthomata *finger pulps* • Osler's nodes & Janeway lesions – *palms*	→ Warm & well perfused or peripherally shut down (CRT>2 sec) → PVD, Raynaud's, CCF or with central cyanosis [↔] → Hypercholesterolaemia → IE [p9 – you could also mention Roth spots here]
Nails	• Finger clubbing (look closely) • Koilonychia • Splinter haemorrhages • Nailfold infarcts	→ IE, cyanotic CHD, atrial myxoma, etc. [p138] → Iron deficiency anaemia → IE, trauma (e.g. gardening, joinery) → Vasculitis, SLE

Wrist	• Radial pulse
	  ○ Rate (time over 15 sec)
	  ○ Rhythm
	  ○ Volume
	  ○ Character
	• Collapsing pulse
	  ○ "Is your shoulder sore at all?"
	  ○ Grasp pt's right wrist with your right hand
	  ○ Place your metacarpal heads over pt's radial artery
	  ○ Support pt's elbow with your left hand
	  ○ Quickly but gently lift their arm up above their head
	• Radio-radial delay (assess over 10 sec)
	• Radio-femoral delay (assess over 10 sec)
		→ Tachycardia / bradycardia
		→ Regular / irregular / irregularly irregular – *AF*
		→ Normal / thready / bounding
		→ Bisferiens pulse (mixed AR/AS), slow rising pulse (AS)
		→ AR
		
		→ A collapsing pulse will thrust against your hand
		→ Cervical rib, aortic coarctation / dissection, embolism
		→ Aortic coarctation / dissection, embolism

Arm	• "I would now measure BP" (in both arms if R-R delay)	→ Pulse pressure (AR wide, AS narrow)
Face	• Malar flush	→ Mitral stenosis
Eyes	• Corneal arcus & xanthelasma • Conjunctival pallor	→ Hypercholesterolaemia → Anaemia
Mouth	• Central cyanosis • Poor dentition	→ Lung disease, cardiac shunt, abnormal Hb [↔] → Risk factor for IE

Neck	• Carotid pulse *volume .*
	  ○ Look for exaggerated pulsation (Corrigan's sign)
	  ○ Briefly palpate
		→ AR
		→ Useful for assessing pulse character; only ever palpate one side at a time

CARDIOVASCULAR

Internal jugular vein on border of SCM.	• JVP	→ [⇨] Causes: P - PE, pericardial ... Q - ↑ Quantity of fluid (overload) R - R sided heart failure S - SVC obstruction. T - Tamponade
	○ Pt at 45°, head turned slightly to right, neck well-lit	→ Don't turn head too far – you want neck muscles to relax
	○ Look for double pulsation on *left* side of neck	→ Easier to see on left as you look *across* pulsation
	○ Estimate height above sternal angle in cm	→ Normally <3–4 cm
	○ *"Do you have a sore stomach at all?"*	
	○ Push on RUQ and watch neck to see JVP rise	→ Normal hepatojugular reflux (increased venous return from liver)
	○ Check JVP rapidly falls back down	→ Persistent elevation of JVP indicates RHF / volume overload

The precordium – remove bra in ♀		
Inspection	• Scars	
	○ Pacemaker / ICD under either clavicle	→ May be an obvious underlying lump – feel if unsure
	○ Midline sternotomy	→ CABG, valve replacement
	○ Left submammary (lift breast to check in ♀)	→ Mitral valvotomy, pericardial window
	○ Legs (if midline sternotomy look now!)	→ Vein harvesting – gives clues to previous surgery [⇨]
	• Visible heave	→ Apical (LVH) or parasternal (RVH)
Palpation (thrills (murmurs), heaves; three hand movements)	• Apex beat	→ Normally in the 5th intercostal space, midclavicular line
	○ Locate & physically count rib spaces	→ If unable to locate, consider why [⇨]
	○ Assess character	→ Tapping (MS), heaving [LVH ΔΔ ⇨], thrusting (MR/AR, LVF)
	• Left parasternal heave	→ Right ventricular hypertrophy
	• Thrills	→ Palpable murmur – grade 4 or above by definition [p9]
Auscultation (*always* whilst palpating carotid pulse – warn pt before doing this)	• 4 primary valve areas	
	○ Apex (Mitral) – **B** then **D**	
	○ LLSE (Tricuspid) – **D**	
	○ 2nd left intercostal space (Pulmonary) – **D**	
	○ 2nd right intercostal space (Aortic) – **D**	
Recommended side of stethoscope **B – Bell** **D – Diaphragm**	• Areas of murmur radiation	
	○ Axilla – **D**	→ MR
	○ Each carotid in turn, breath held in expiration – **D**	→ AS (hold your breath too so you know when pt must breathe)
	• Manoeuvres to amplify diastolic murmurs	
	○ Apex, pt on LHS, breath held in expiration – **B**	→ Amplifies MS (note also tends to amplify MR)
	○ LLSE, pt sitting forward, breath held in expiration – **D**	→ Amplifies AR (note also tends to amplify AS)

Back	• Auscultate lung bases for crepitations	→ LHF
	• Palpate for sacral oedema	→ RHF
Ankles	• Peripheral oedema	→ RHF, numerous other causes [p139]

Conclusion	• Wash / gel hands, thank pt & allow to re-dress	
	• Review observation chart (HR, BP, RR, SpO_2, temperature)	
	• Abdominal examination & peripheral pulses	→ Hepatomegaly & ascites (RHF), splenomegaly (IE), AAA
	• Investigations: ECG, CXR, echocardiogram, urinalysis	→ Microscopic haematuria (IE)

Cardiac surgery scars give you clues during examination
- Midline sternotomy + leg scar = simple CABG most likely, possible valve replacement with CABG
- Midline sternotomy with no leg scar = valve replacement most likely, possible CABG without vein graft (LIMA or radial artery graft only)

Key JVP abnormalities
- Elevated — RHF, volume overload, PE, constrictive pericarditis
- Elevated with ↓BP — Tension pneumothorax, cardiac tamponade, massive PE, severe asthma
- Elevated & fixed — SVC obstruction
- Cannon A waves — Complete heart block, VEBs, VT
- Giant V waves — TR (look for ear-wiggling, feel for pulsatile hepatomegaly)

Differentiating between types of cyanosis
- Pure peripheral cyanosis causes *cold* blue hands
- Central cyanosis causes blue lips and tongue, and when severe can also cause blue hands (usually *warm*)

ΔΔ Central cyanosis (blue lips & tongue)
- Hypoxic lung disease
- Right-to-left cardiac shunt
  - Cyanotic congenital heart disease
  - Eisenmenger's syndrome
- Methaemoglobinaemia
  - Drugs
  - Toxins

ΔΔ Irregularly irregular pulse
- AF
- Ventricular ectopic beats (VEBs)
- Complete HB + variable ventricular escape

To differentiate between AF and VEBs without an ECG you can exercise the pt – this will abolish VEBs but AF will remain

Six important causes of AF
- Ischaemic heart disease
- Rheumatic heart disease
- Thyrotoxicosis
- Pneumonia
- PE
- Alcohol

ΔΔ Peripheral cyanosis (blue hands)
- Peripheral vascular disease
- Raynaud's syndrome
- Heart failure
- Shock
- (Central cyanosis when severe)

Some causes of an absent radial pulse
- Congenital (usually bilateral)
- Arterial embolism (e.g. due to AF)
- Atheroma (usually subclavian)
- Previous arterial line
- Previous coronary angiography
- Cervical rib
- Coarctation of the aorta

Features of the JVP (vs carotid pulse)
- Double pulsation
- Non-palpable
- Obliterated when pressure applied at base of neck
- Height changes with respiration
- Height changes with angle of pt
- Rises with hepatojugular reflux

Pulsus paradoxus
- An exaggeration of the normal situation in which BP falls during inspiration, to such an extent that during inspiration the peripheral pulse may not be felt despite the LV contracting (and heart sounds still being heard)
- Causes: tamponade, constrictive pericarditis, restrictive cardiomyopathy, severe asthma / COPD

Kussmaul's sign
- A rise in the JVP on inspiration, which is the opposite of normal (due to impaired RV filling)
- Causes: tamponade, constrictive pericarditis, restrictive cardiomyopathy

Causes of a non-palpable apex beat
1. Something is between your fingers and the apex
   - Adipose tissue (obese pt)
   - Air (pneuothorax or emphysema)
   - Fluid (pleural or pericardial effusion)
2. The apex is not in its normal position
   - Displaced (usually laterally in LHF)
   - Dextrocardia

CCF = biventricular failure = LHF + RHF

ΔΔ Heaving apex (LVH)
- Aortic stenosis
- Hypertension
- HOCM
- Coarctation of the aorta

CXR features of LHF (ABCDE)
- Alveolar oedema
- Kerley **B** lines
- **C**ardiomegaly
- Upper lobe venous **D**iversion
- Pleural **E**ffusion

Causes of pericarditis
- Viral (Coxsackie)
- Bacterial / fungal infection
- Immediately post-MI
- Dressler's syndrome (2–10 weeks post-MI)
- SLE / RA / scleroderma
- Uraemia
- Malignancy

3rd heart sound
- Due to rapid ventricular filling
- May be normal if <30 years old
- Think *volume overload*
- Causes: CCF, MR, AR, large anterior MI

4th heart sound
- Due to poorly compliant ventricle
- Always abnormal
- Cannot occur in AF (requires atrial systole)
- Think *pressure overload*
- Causes: AS, HTN, HOCM, post-MI fibrosis

Causes of cardiac failure
1. Pump failure
   - IHD
   - Cardiomyopathy
   - Constrictive pericarditis
   - Arrhythmia
   - Drugs (negative inotropes)
2. Excessive preload
   - Regurgitant valvular disease (MR / AR)
   - Fluid overload (renal failure, IV fluids)
   - VSD
3. Excessive afterload
   - AS
   - HTN
4. High-output failure (rare)
   - Anaemia
   - Pregnancy
   - Metabolic (hyperthyroidism, Paget's)
5. Isolated RHF
   - Cor pulmonale
   - Primary pulmonary HTN

CARDIOVASCULAR NOTES

		Mitral stenosis	Mitral regurgitation

Aetiology		• Rheumatic heart disease (99%)	• Primary MR (structural)
			  ○ Rheumatic heart disease
			  ○ IE
			  ○ Valve prolapse
			  ○ Papillary muscle rupture (e.g. post-MI)
			  ○ Marfan's
			  ○ SLE
			• Secondary MR (functional)
			  ○ LV dilatation

Presentation		• SOB & fatigue • Pulmonary oedema / haemoptysis • RHF (late)	• SOB & fatigue • Other LVF (orthopnoea, PND)
Features [⇨]	T	• Mid-diastolic	• Pansystolic
	I	• 1–4	• 1–6
	P	• Apex	• Apex
	P	• On LHS & with expiration (bell)	• –
	Q	• Rumbling (low-pitched)	• Blowing
	R	• None	• Axilla
	S	• Opening snap • Tapping apex • AF • Loud 1st heart sound • Mitral facies • Signs of RHF (late)	• 3rd heart sound • Thrusting, displaced apex • Quiet 1st heart sound • Obliterated 2nd heart sound • AF • Audible 'click' in valve prolapse
ECG features		• AF common • P mitrale (bifid P waves)	• AF common • VEBs
CXR features		• Enlarged left atrium • Pulmonary venous congestion	• Cardiomegaly (late) • Cardiac failure [p5]

ΔΔ		• Austin Flint (2° AR)
		• Carey Coombs (rheumatic fever)
		• TS (usually rheumatic)
			• VSD (important ΔΔ post-MI)
			• TR (usually functional)
			  ○ Pulsatile hepatomegaly
			  ○ Giant V waves in JVP
			• AS (in ΔΔ for any systolic murmur)

Medical Rx		• AF Rx + anticoagulation • Diuretics	• AF Rx + anticoagulation • Diuretics • ACEi (HTN worsens MR)

Common indications for surgery (*Eur Heart J*, 2012; 33: 2451)		• Moderate / severe disease
		• Percutaneous balloon valvuloplasty usually preferred technique
		• Contraindications to percutaneous technique (therefore perform open repair / replacement)
		  ○ Persistent LA thrombus
		  ○ Moderate / severe MR
		  ○ Rigid calcified valve
		  ○ Pt requires CABG anyway
			• Severe primary disease, plus
			  ○ Symptoms, or
			  ○ LV impairment / dilatation (but do not delay until irreversible structural damage occurs)
			• Valve repair usually preferable over replacement
			• Surgery for secondary MR is controversial

HEART MURMURS

		Aortic stenosis	Aortic regurgitation
Aetiology		• Rheumatic heart disease • Calcified bicuspid valve (age 50–60) • Calcified tricuspid valve (age 70+)	• Rheumatic heart disease • IE • Luetic heart disease (syphilis) • Bicuspid valve • Hypertension • Aortic dissection • Marfan's • RA • Ankylosing spondylitis
Presentation		1. SOB 2. Syncope / pre-syncope } Classic OSCE questions 3. Angina	• SOB & fatigue • Palpitations • (Often asymptomatic)
Features [⇨]	T	• Ejection systolic	• Early diastolic
	I	• 1–6	• 1–4
	P	• Aortic	• LLSE
	P	• –	• Sitting up & with expiration (diaphragm)
	Q	• Crescendo–decrescendo	• Breath-like (high-pitched)
	R	• Carotids	• None
	S	• 4th heart sound • Heaving apex • Slow-rising pulse • Narrow pulse pressure • Ejection click • Quiet 2nd heart sound (if severe)	• 3rd heart sound • Thrusting, displaced apex • Collapsing pulse • Wide pulse pressure • Eponymous signs [⇨] • Austin Flint murmur (mid-diastolic)
ECG features		• LVH / LV strain pattern	–
CXR features		–	• Cardiomegaly • Cardiac failure [p4]
ΔΔ		• Aortic sclerosis [⇨] • HOCM • PS (usually congenital) • MR (in ΔΔ for any systolic murmur)	• PR • Graham Steele (PR 2° pulmonary hypertension)
Medical Rx		Treat HTN	• Diuretics • Vasodilators

Common indications for surgery (Eur Heart J, 2012; 33: 2451)		• Severe disease, plus
		  ○ Symptoms, or
		  ○ LV impairment
		• Moderate / severe disease and undergoing CABG or other valve surgery
		• Intervention in asymptomatic severe AS remains controversial
		• TAVI if unfit for open surgery
		• Valvuloplasty becoming rarer (may be used as interim measure prior to TAVI)
			• Severe disease, plus
			  ○ Symptoms, or
			  ○ LV impairment / dilatation (but do not delay until irreversible structural damage occurs)

HEART MURMURS

System for describing features of a heart murmur

It can be difficult to recall the features of a murmur. To help do this, use a method such as the TIPPQRS system. Keep reciting T-I-P-P-Q-R-S to yourself until it comes instantly.

T   Timing
I   Intensity – thrills are rare so generally grade 2 if quiet and grade 3 if loud
     (if you say grade 1 you are claiming to be an expert!)
P_1 Position of stethoscope on precordium where heard loudest
P_2 Position of pt when murmur heard loudest – usually only relevant to diastolic murmurs
Q   Quality
R   Radiation
S   Systemic features – other heart sounds, characteristics of the apex beat / pulse, etc.

How to present your findings

Go through TIPPQRS

* On auscultation, the 1st & 2nd heart sounds are normal / loud / quiet / prosthetic / not heard
* There is a $\boxed{T}$ murmur of grade $\boxed{I}$ intensity heard loudest in the $\boxed{P_1}$ area with the pt $\boxed{P_2}$
* The murmur is $\boxed{Q}$ in nature and radiates to the $\boxed{R}$ (or does not radiate)
* There is an associated $\boxed{S}$ (3rd/4th heart sounds, apex beat & pulse characteristics, etc.)
* In summary my findings on examination fit with a diagnosis of _____
* List the differential diagnosis if appropriate
* If native valves: there are no stigmata of IE or signs of heart failure (if you have checked!)
* If prosthetic valve: there is no evidence of valve failure or IE

Example 1: On auscultation, the 1st and 2nd heart sounds are normal. There is an early diastolic murmur of grade 2 intensity heard loudest at the lower left sternal edge with the pt sitting forward and breath held in expiration. The murmur is high-pitched and breath-like in nature and does not radiate. There is an associated 3rd heart sound, a thrusting apex beat and a collapsing pulse. In summary, my findings on examination fit with a diagnosis of aortic regurgitation. There are no apparent stigmata of infective endocarditis or signs of heart failure.

Example 2: On auscultation, a normal 1st heart sound is audible with a prosthetic 2nd heart sound. There is an associated ejection systolic murmur of grade 3 intensity heard loudest in the aortic area. The murmur has a crescendo–decrescendo quality and radiates to both carotids. This is likely to be a flow murmur across a prosthetic aortic valve. There is no evidence of valvular complication, particularly valve failure or IE.

HEART MURMURS NOTES

By far the most common murmurs in OSCEs are AS and MR, but AR does pop up pretty frequently so *always* palpate the carotid pulse when auscultating and decide if the murmur occurs with the pulse (i.e. systolic) or between pulses (i.e. diastolic). Remember left-sided murmurs are louder on expiration, right-sided murmurs on inspiration.

Grading of murmur intensity
- Grade 1   Very faint, just audible by an expert in optimal conditions
- Grade 2   Quiet, just audible by a non-expert in optimal conditions
- Grade 3   Moderately loud
- Grade 4   Loud with palpable thrill
- Grade 5   Very loud with thrill, audible with stethoscope partly off chest ⎤
- Grade 6   Very loud with thrill, audible without a stethoscope   ⎦ Systolic only

Stigmata of infective endocarditis
- Changing heart murmurs
- Finger clubbing
- Splinter haemorrhages
- Mild splenomegaly
- Microscopic haematuria
- Eponymous signs (rare!)
  - Osler's nodes on finger pulps
  - Janeway lesions on palms and soles
  - Roth spots on the retina

Complications of prosthetic valves
- Structural valve failure*
- Paravalvular leak*
- Thrombosis & obstruction
- Infective endocarditis
- Intravascular haemolysis
- (Warfarin-related complications)

*Both cause regurgitant murmurs

Aortic 'sclerosis'
- *Asymptomatic*
- Does not radiate to carotids
- No slow-rising pulse
- Normal pulse pressure
- 2nd heart sound normal / loud

Eponymous signs in AR
- Corrigan's: Exaggerated carotid pulse
- Quinke's: Nailbed pulsation
- De Musset's: Head-nodding
- Duroziez's: Diastolic femoral murmur
- Traube's: 'Pistol shot' femorals

Indications for a bioprosthetic valve
(do not require warfarinisation but only last 10–15 years)
1. Elderly
   (if you predict that valve will outlast pt)
2. Contraindication to warfarin
   (e.g. Woman of childbearing age – considered on a case-by-case basis, weighing up against need to re-replace valve in future)
3. Patient choice
   (once adequately informed)

	Action / Examine for	ΔΔ / Potential findings / Extra information
Introduction	• Wash / gel hands • Introduce yourself, confirm pt, explain examination & gain consent • Expose & position pt (top off), supine at 45°)	→ Consider chaperone → If only examining posterior chest, sit on side of bed now
End of the bed	• General appearance – well / unwell / distressed / dyspnoeic • Accessory muscle use, pursed-lip breathing • Nutritional status / cachexia • Oxygen, fluids and medications • *Look inside sputum pot if available*	→ Pursed lip breathing = lower airway obstruction (usually COPD) → COPD, malignancy → Inhalers & nebulisers especially → Describe colour, purulence, presence of blood, etc.
Hands	• Peripheral cyanosis • Feel temperature • Dilated veins • Tar staining / coal dust tattoos • 1st web space wasting	→ PVD, Raynaud's, CCF or with central cyanosis [p4] → Central cyanosis = warm, pure peripheral cyanosis = cold [p4] → Hypercapnia → Smoking / mining (risk of coal-worker's pneumoconiosis) → T_1 lesion (e.g. Pancoast tumour)
Nails	• Finger clubbing (look closely) • Koilonychia	→ Ca, ILD, suppurative lung disease, etc. [p138] → Iron deficiency anaemia (cause of SOB)

Wrist	• Flapping tremor (asterixis)
	• Fine physiological tremor
	• Respiratory rate
	• Radial pulse
	  ○ Rate
	  ○ Volume
		→ Respiratory failure (CO_2 retention), hepatic / renal failure
		→ β_2-agonist Rx (e.g. Salbutamol)
		→ Count over 15 sec whilst pretending to take pulse
		
		→ Tachycardia if unwell, distressed, on β_2-agonist Rx
		→ Bounding in hypercapnia

Face	• Cushingoid (moon face, plethora, acne, hirsute)	→ Long-term steroid Rx (e.g. for CFA), others [p84]
Eyes	• Conjunctival pallor • Horner's (ptosis, miosis)	→ Anaemia (cause of SOB) → Pancoast tumour [↔]
Mouth	• Central cyanosis • Candida	→ Hypoxic lung disease, cardiac shunt, abnormal Hb [p4] → Steroid inhalers, immunocompromised pt

Neck	• JVP [p3 for technique]
	• Trachea
	  ○ *"I'm going to feel for your windpipe"*
	  ○ Position
	  ○ Cricosternal distance
	  ○ *"Take a deep breath in"*
	  ○ Tug on inspiration
	• Lymph nodes
	  ○ *"Do you have any pain in your neck?"*
	  ○ Palpate systematically [p136 for technique]
		→ Elevated in RHF, PE, SVC obstruction, etc. [p4]
		
		→ Always warm the pt before doing this
		→ Deviates towards collapse, away from tension / big effusion
		→ Normally 2–3 fingers, reduced in hyperinflation (COPD)
		
		→ Hyperinflation (COPD)
		
		→ Tender = infection, non-tender = suspicious of malignancy

RESPIRATORY

sternotomy —

The chest
anterior chest with pt supine at 45°, then repeat on posterior chest with pt sitting on side of bed, arms crossed in front to separate scapulae

Inspection	• A–P diameter	→ Hyperinflation (COPD)
	• Scars (check carefully around the sides & back)	→ Thoracotomy (lobectomy / pneumonectomy), old chest drain sites,
	• Deformity of chest / spine	→ Pectus excavatum, pectus carinatum (asthma), scoliosis
	• Intercostal indrawing (*Hoover's sign*)	→ Hyperinflation (COPD)
Palpation	• Chest expansion	
	○ *"Take deep breaths in and out"*	→ Large degree of asymmetry may be obvious on inspection
	○ Watch chest wall movement first	→ Assess symmetry rather than degree of expansion (hard to quantify)
	○ Palpate chest wall in 2 separate places	
	• Apex beat (particularly lateral / medial displacement)	→ Mediastinal shift (collapse, tension, big effusion)
	• RV heave	→ RVH (possible cor pulmonale)
Percussion	• Assess percussion note	→ Resonant, dull, stony dull [⇔]
	○ Start in supraclavicular fossae & work down chest	→ 8–10 places is usually sufficient
	○ Compare side to side, including axillae	
	○ Map out any abnormalities	
Auscultation (Diaphragm unless very hairy or skinny)	• Breath sounds & added noises	[⇔]
	○ *"Take deep breaths in and out through your mouth"*	→ Specifying mouth avoids noisy nasal breathing
	○ Same sequence as for percussion	→ 8–10 places is usually sufficient
	○ Listen for breath sound presence & character	→ Character can be vesicular or bronchial (consolidation)
	○ Wheeze	→ Small airway obstruction (asthma, COPD)
	○ Crepitations	→ Fluid in airspaces: secretions, pus, oedema
	○ If crepitations heard, ask pt to cough & listen again	→ If due to normal secretions, crepitations should clear with cough
	• Vocal resonance	→ ↑ in consolidation, ↓ in collapse / effusion / pneumothorax
	○ *"Say 99 each time I put my stethoscope on your chest"*	→ 8–10 places is usually sufficient
	○ Same sequence as for percussion	→ Loud conduction of whispered voice due to consolidation
	• Whispering pectoriloquy	
	○ *"Now whisper 99 each time I touch your chest"*	
	○ Check only in areas of ↑ VR or bronchial breathing	

Back	• Sacral oedema	→ RHF
Ankles	• Peripheral oedema	→ RHF (e.g. cor pulmonale), multiple other causes [p139]

Conclusion	• Wash / gel hands, thank pt & allow to re-dress
	• See sputum pot (if not already seen)
	• Review observation chart (HR, BP, RR, SpO_2, temperature)
	• Investigations: Peak flow, PFTs, CXR, ABG

RESPIRATORY

How to present your findings

Work through the examination sequence

- The pt was [dyspnoeic / comfortable] at rest breathing [air / O_2], and [cyanosed / not cyanosed]
- The respiratory rate was _____ breaths per minute
- Always comment on clubbing, lymphadenopathy and mediastinal shift
- List any other peripheral signs found
- Comment on expansion, percussion, breath sounds, added sounds, vocal resonance
- Give differential diagnosis
- Comment on the presence / absence of cor pulmonale if chronic lung disease (COPD, ILD)

Example: The pt was dyspnoeic at rest breathing air, and centrally cyanosed. The respiratory rate was 25 breaths per min. There was finger clubbing but no lymphadenopathy or mediastinal shift. Chest expansion was symmetrical and the percussion note resonant throughout. Breath sounds were present throughout the chest and vesicular. In addition fine inspiratory crepitations were heard bibasally. Vocal resonance was normal. The differential diagnosis includes interstitial lung disease and pulmonary oedema.

	Consolidation	Collapse*	Effusion**	Pneumothorax	Pneumonectomy
Mediastinal shift	–	Towards	Away if big	Away if tension	Towards
Percussion note	Dull	Dull	Stony dull	(Hyper) resonant	Dull
Breath sounds	Bronchial or ↓	↓ or absent	↓ or absent	↓ or absent	Absent
Vocal resonance	←	↓ or absent	↓ or absent	↓ or absent	Absent

***Lobectomy / pneumonectomy**
- Examination findings identical to collapse
- Given away by thoracotomy scar on chest, but some examiners will hide this to test you
- Indications: Bronchogenic Ca (25% of non-SCLC is resectable), bronchiectasis, trauma, TB

****Raised hemidiaphragm**
- Examination findings identical to effusion
- CXR to differentiate
- Due to phrenic nerve palsy
- Caused by thoracic surgery / trauma / malignancy

Signs of hyperinflation
- Reduced cricosternal distance ± tracheal tug
- Increased A–P diameter
- Intercostal indrawing (Hoover's sign)
- Apex beat not palpable
- Hyper-resonant percussion note

ΔΔ Interstitial lung disease (pulmonary fibrosis)

1. Idiopathic
   - Cryptogenic fibrosing alveolitis
2. Due to inhaled antigen (i.e. EAA)
   - Bird fancier's lung
   - Farmer's lung
3. Due to inhaled irritant
   - Asbestosis
   - Silicosis
   - Coal worker's pneumoconiosis
4. Associated with systemic disease
   - SLE
   - RA
   - Sarcoid
   - Systemic sclerosis
5. Iatrogenic
   - Methotrexate
   - Amiodarone
   - Radiotherapy

ΔΔ Horner's syndrome

- Central lesion
   - Stroke / tumour / MS
   - Syringobulbia
- T_1 root lesion
   - Spondylosis
   - Neurofibroma
- Brachial plexus lesion
   - Pancoast tumour
   - Cervical rib
   - Trauma / birth injury (Klumpke's)
- Neck lesion
   - Tumour
   - Carotid artery aneurysm
   - Sympathectomy
- With cluster headaches

Features of bronchial breathing

- Loud and blowing   = high pitch .
- Length of inspiration = expiration
- Audible gap between inspiration & expiration
- Reproducible by placing your stethoscope over your own trachea and listening

ΔΔ Bibasal crepitations

- Fine
   - Pulmonary oedema
   - Interstitial lung disease
- Coarse
   - Bronchiectesis
   - Cystic fibrosis
   - Bibasal pneumonia

ΔΔ Pleural effusion

- Transudate (Protein <30 g/l)
   - LVF
   - Volume overload
   - Hypoalbuminaemia [p139]
   - Meig's syndrome
- Exudate (protein >30 g/l)
   - Infection
      - Pneumonia
      - TB
   - Infarction
      - PE
   - Inflammation
      - RA
      - SLE
   - Malignancy
      - Bronchogenic
      - Mesothelioma

NOTES

Bronchial breath sounds are abnormal over lung fields - heard in trachea

Vesicular - lower pitched, should be normal.

Bronchial suggests - consolidation, tension pneumothorax, massive pleural effusion

	Action / Examine for	ΔΔ / Potential findings / Extra information
Introduction	• Wash / gel hands • Introduce yourself, confirm pt, explain examination & gain consent • Expose pt (xiphisternum to pubic symphysis) • Position pt (supine at 45°) • *"Do you have any pain in your tummy? If so, where?"*	→ Consider chaperone → Traditional 'nipples to knees' exposure is rarely necessary → Do not lie flat yet
End of the bed	• General appearance – well / unwell / distressed / in pain • Oxygen, drips, catheters, medications, drains • Nutritional status / cachexia	→ Wasting due to malabsorption or synthetic liver failure
Hands	• Tendon xanthomata • Dupuytren's contracture – *feel* palm for this • Palmar erythema	→ Hyperlipidaemia (PBC, cholestasis) → CLD, diabetes, heavy labour, phenytoin, trauma, familial → CLD, pregnancy, hyperthyroidism, RA
Nails	• Finger clubbing (look closely) • Leuconychia • Koilonychia	→ IBD, cirrhosis, lymphoma, coeliac disease, etc. [p138] → Hypoalbuminaemia (CLD, other causes) [p139] → Iron-deficiency anaemia (e.g. GI bleeding)
Wrist	• Flapping tremor (*asterixis*) • Radial pulse rate – palpate briefly	→ Hepatic failure (encephalopathy), respiratory / renal failure → Quick assessment of circulatory status
Arms	• Bruising • IVDU marks	→ CLD (due to thombocytopaenia, clotting factors, falls) → Risk of hepatitis B & C
Face	• Cushingoid (moon face, plethora, acne, hirsute) • Parotid enlargement (*sialoadenosis*)	→ Alcohol excess (alcoholic pseudo-Cushing's), others [p84] → Alcohol excess
Eyes	• Scleral icterus • Corneal arcus & xanthelasma • Episcleritis / conjunctivitis • Conjunctival pallor	→ Jaundice (implies serum bilirubin >35 μmol/l) → Hyperlipidaemia (PBC, cholestasis) → Associated with IBD [⇔] → Anaemia
Mouth	• Angular stomatitis & glossitis (large, smooth tongue) • Oral candidiasis • Apthous ulcers • Fetor hepaticus (musty, sweet breath odour)	→ Iron / folate / B$_{12}$ deficiency → Immunodeficiency → IBD (especially Crohn's) → Hepatic failure (mercaptan accumulation)

Neck	• Lymph nodes
	  ○ *"Do you have any pain in your neck?"*
	  ○ Palpate systematically [p137 for technique]
		→ Virchow's node = left supraclavicular (e.g. gastric Ca)

Chest / Back	• Gynaecomastia • Loss of secondary sexual hair • Spider naevi – *depress* to demonstrate central filling	→ CLD, drugs, testicular failure, etc. [⇔] → CLD → Occur in distribution of SVC, ⩾5 suggests CLD

The abdomen – lie flat with one pillow & arms resting at sides to relax musculature

Inspection	• Abdominal distension	→ The 6 Fs: **F**at, **F**luid, **F**latus, **F**aeces, **F**etus, **F**ecking big masses
	• Caput medusa (dilated veins from umbilicus outwards)	→ Portal hypertension
	• Scars	→ Numerous types [↻]
Palpation (and a little percussion)	• General palpation	→ Tenderness, guarding, masses
	○ Get down on one knee, keep watching pt's face	→ Watching the face is key; examiners will scrutinise you for it
	○ *"Tell me if I cause you any discomfort"*	
	○ Start furthest away from any tender area	→ Keep watching the pt's face!
	○ Work round 9 areas, light then deep palpation	→ Hepatomegaly [↻]
	• Liver	
	○ *"Take deep breaths in and out"*	
	○ Start in RIF, work up towards right costal margin	→ Liver edge will flick under your fingers as it descends
	○ Feel for liver edge during *inspiration*	→ Percuss down from axilla to find upper border
	○ Percuss out upper & lower hepatic borders	→ Splenomegaly [↻]
	• Spleen	→ [p20: differentiating between spleen & left kidney]
	○ *"Take deep breaths in and out"*	→ As for liver, feel during inspiration
	○ Start in RIF, work up towards left costal margin	→ Encourages an enlarged spleen to come out from behind ribs
	○ If not felt, repeat with pt on RHS and your left hand gently pulling pt's left lower ribs forward	
	• Kidneys – ballot each in turn	→ [p20: ΔΔ unilateral / bilateral enlarged kidneys]
	• AAA – palpate deeply with 2 hands above umbilicus	→ Do this *very* briefly unless specifically instructed – not technically GI but cause of abdominal symptoms
Percussion	• Shifting dullness	→ Ascites (usually ≥1.5 l of fluid present if shifting dullness) [↻]
	○ Percuss away from midline towards left flank	→ Avoids hepatic dullness on the right
	○ Leave finger at first point of dullness	
	○ Roll pt towards you	
	○ Percuss again – if now tympanic test is +ve	→ Fluid (& dullness) shifts with gravity
Auscultation	• Bowel sounds – just below umbilicus (1 min max)	→ Active, sluggish, tinkling / obstructive
	• Renal bruits – superior and lateral to umbilicus	→ Renal artery disease
	• Liver bruit if liver edge felt	→ HCC, AV malformation, TIPSS

Legs	• Peripheral oedema	→ CLD, multiple other causes [p139]
	• Erythema nodosum	→ IBD [p97 for ΔΔ]
	• Pyoderma gangrenosum	→ IBD, RA

Conclusion	• Wash / gel hands, thank pt & allow them to re-dress	
	• Examine groins, genitalia & perform digital rectal examination [p118]	→ Groin herniae, testicular atrophy in CLD
	• Review observation chart (HR, BP, RR, SpO₂, temperature)	

GASTROINTESTINAL

Abdominal scars

1. Kocher's (subcostal) – open cholecystectomy
2. Right paramedian laparotomy – various (e.g. pancreatic transplant)
3. Midline laparotomy
4. Nephrectomy
5. Gridiron – appendicectomy
6. Laparoscopic – various (cholecystectomy, appendectomy, gynae procedures)
7. Left paramedian – anterior resection of rectum
8. Pfannenstiel / transverse suprapubic – TAH, Caesarian section

Multifactorial aetiology of ascites in CLD

1. Portal hypertension
2. Hypoalbuminaemia
3. Salt & water retention 2° RAAS activation

ΔΔ Ascites – compare with ΔΔ pleural effusion

- Transudate (protein <30 g/l)
  - CLD (75% of ascites)
  - RHF
  - Volume overload
  - Hypoalbuminaemia [p139]
  - Constrictive pericarditis
- Exudate (protein >30 g/l)
  - Infection
    - SBP
    - TB
  - Inflammation
    - Pancreatitis
  - Malignancy
    - Luminal (stomach / colon)
    - Pancreas
    - Liver (primary / metastatic)
    - Ovarian
    - Lymphoma

ΔΔ Hepatomegaly

Remember the categories: 2 Is, 2 Bs & 2 Cs

- **Infection**
  - Viral hepatitis*
  - EBV*
  - Malaria*
  - Hepatic abscess
- **Infiltration**
  - Sarcoid*
  - Amyloid*
  - Fatty liver
  - Haemochromatosis
- **Blood-related**
  - Lymphoma*
  - Leukaemia*
  - Myeloproliferative disorders*
  - Haemolytic anaemias*
- **Biliary**
  - PBC
  - PSC
- **Cancer**
  - Primary HCC
  - Metastatic deposits
- **Congestion**
  - RHF
  - Tricuspid regurgitation
  - Budd–Chiari syndrome

*Important causes of hepatosplenomegaly – a tricky list which you should know for exams

GASTROINTESTINAL NOTES

Extra-intestinal manifestations of IBD
- Finger clubbing
- Mouth ulcers (especially Crohn's)
- Eyes:
  - Episcleritis
  - Conjunctivitis
- Skin:
  - Erythema nodosum
  - Pyoderma gangrenosum
- Joints: Seronegative spondyloarthropathy
- PSC (especially UC)
- Amyloidosis (especially Crohn's)

ΔΔ Gynaecomastia
- Physiological (puberty / elderly)
- Testicular failure
  - Klinefelter's syndrome
  - Viral orchitis / testicular trauma
  - Haemodialysis
- Increased oestrogen
  - Chronic liver disease
  - Thyrotoxicosis
  - Oestrogen-secreting tumour
- Drug-induced (e.g. digoxin, isoniazid, spiro)

Liver edge characteristics
- Smooth
  - Venous congestion
  - Fatty infiltration
- Knobbly
  - Metastases
  - Cysts
- Pulsatile
  - Tricuspid regurgitation
- Tender
  - Hepatitis
  - RHF (capsular pain)
- Bruit
  - HCC
  - AV malformation
  - TIPSS

Causes of Massive splenomegaly (past umbilicus)
- Malaria
- Myelofibrosis
- CML

Other important causes of splenomegaly
- Infective endocarditis
- RA (if low WCC this is Felty's syndrome)

A note on portal hypertension
- Does not cause hepatomegaly
- Does cause splenomegaly
- When associated with early hepatic disease (e.g. chronic active hepatitis) which itself causes hepatomegaly, the overall result may be hepatosplenomegaly
- When associated with relatively late hepatic disease (e.g. cirrhosis) which causes a shrunken liver, the overall result is isolated splenomegaly
- Also causes caput medusae, oesophageal varices, gastropathy & ascites

	Action / Examine for	ΔΔ / Potential findings / Extra information
Introduction	• Wash / gel hands • Introduce yourself, confirm pt, explain examination & gain consent • Expose pt (xiphisternum to pubic symphysis) • Position pt (supine at 45°) • *"Do you have any pain in your tummy? If so, where?"*	→ Consider chaperone → Traditional 'nipples to knees' exposure is rarely necessary → Do not lie flat yet
End of the bed	• General appearance – well / unwell / distressed / in pain • Oxygen, drips, catheters, medications, drains • Nutritional status / cachexia	→ Chronic illness / malignancy
Wrists	• Flapping tremor (*asterixis*) • Radial pulse rate – palpate briefly	→ Renal failure, hepatic / respiratory failure → Quick assessment of circulatory status

Arms	• Look for AV fistula
	  ○ Wrist
	  ○ Antecubital fossa
	• Examine AV fistula if present
	  ○ Palpate for thrill
	  ○ Auscultate for loud bruit
	• Parathyroid implantation scar
	  ○ Wrist
	  ○ Shoulder
	• *"I would now measure BP"*
		→ Radio-cephalic ('Cimino') fistula
		→ Brachio-cephalic or brachio-basilic fistula
		→ You may be asked to examine this as a 'lump' [p94]
		→ Due to turbulent flow – absent if fistula thrombosed
		→ As above
		→ Parathyroid tissue implanted following parathyroidectomy
		
		→ Never measure BP on fistula arm

Face / Eyes	• Conjunctival pallor • Yellow tinge to skin	→ Anaemia (common in CRF: chronic disease, epo deficiency) → Uraemia (ΔΔ jaundice)

Neck	• JVP [p3 for technique]
	• Central venous catheter
	  ○ Current
	  ○ Scar from previous CV catheter at base of neck
	• Parathyroidectomy scar
		→ Fluid overload
		
		→ Usually a transverse scar on lower neck

CHRONIC RENAL FAILURE / RENAL TRANSPLANT

The abdomen – lie flat with one pillow & arms resting at sides to relax musculature

Inspection	• Abdominal distension	→ The 6 Fs: Fat, Fluid, Flatus, Faeces, Fetus, Fecking big masses (including polycystic kidneys)
	• Tenckhoff catheter (peritoneal dialysis)	
	○ Current	
	○ Scar from previous near umbilicus	
	• Nephrectomy scars	→ Check flanks
	• Renal transplant scars	→ Right / left iliac fossa (unless pt is Jonah Lomu). *look very carefully*
Palpation	• General palpation	→ Tenderness, guarding, masses
	○ Get down on one knee, keep watching pt's face	→ Watching the face is key; examiners will scrutinise you for it
	○ *"Tell me if I cause you any discomfort"*	
	○ Start furthest away from any tender area	→ Keep watching the pt's face!
	○ Work round 9 areas, light then deep palpation	→ Unilateral / bilateral enlargement [⇔]
	• Kidneys	
	○ Ballot flanks for each kidney in turn	→ [⇕]
	○ Differentiate left kidney from spleen if necessary	
	• Transplanted kidney	→ Sometimes difficult to palpate
	○ Palpate for this under LIF/RIF scar	
	• Liver	→ Polycystic hepatomegaly can occur in APKD
	○ Palpate if kidneys enlarged [p15 for technique]	
Percussion	• Shifting dullness if Tenckhoff catheter *in situ*	→ Ascites (in this case peritoneal dialysate)
	○ Percuss away from midline towards left flank	→ Avoids hepatic dullness on the right
	○ Leave finger at first point of dullness	
	○ Roll pt towards you	
	○ Percuss again – if now tympanic test is +ve	→ Fluid (& dullness) shifts with gravity
Auscultation	• Renal bruits – superior and lateral to umbilicus	→ Renal artery disease

Back	• Auscultate lung bases for crepitations	→ Fluid overload
	• Palpate for sacral oedema	→ Fluid overload
Ankles	• Ankle oedema	→ Fluid overload [p139]

Conclusion	• Wash / gel hands, thank pt & allow them to re-dress	
	• Review observation chart (HR, BP, RR, SpO_2, temperature)	
	• Investigations: urinalysis, renal USS	→ May shed light on aetiology of CRF

CHRONIC RENAL FAILURE / RENAL TRANSPLANT

ΔΔ LIF mass
- Renal transplant
- Loaded colon
- Diverticular mass
- Colorectal carcinoma
- Ovarian mass / cyst

ΔΔ Bilateral enlarged kidneys
- APKD
- Bilateral hydronephrosis
- Amyloidosis

ΔΔ Unilateral enlarged kidney
- Hydronephrosis
- Renal cancer
- Renal cyst

Indications for dialysis in CRF
- Progressive decline in renal function (usually CKD Stage 5 = GFR <15 ml/min)
- Symptomatic uraemia despite conservative Rx
- Renal bone disease
- Pericarditis
- Volume overload despite fluid restriction & diuretics
- Hyperkalaemia despite Rx

ΔΔ RIF mass
- Renal transplant
- Appendix mass
- Crohn's disease (inflamed, matted small intestine)
- Caecal carcinoma
- Ovarian mass / cyst

Spleen versus left kidney on examination
- You can get your hand over a kidney
- Percussion note is resonant over a kidney
- Kidney is ballottable
- Spleen has a notch
- Spleen moves more on respiration

NOTES

CHRONIC RENAL FAILURE/RENAL TRANSPLANT NOTES

Aspects of renal bone disease

1. Osteomalacia due to vitamin D deficiency
2. Hyperparathyroidism due to ↑ serum phosphate
   - Subperiosteal bone resorption, especially on hand X-ray
   - Pepper pot skull (ΔΔ multiple myeloma)
3. Osteosclerosis due to prolonged hyperparathyroidism
   - 'Rugger jersey' spine
4. Osteoporosis

Complications of haemodialysis

- Hypotension
- Hypovolaemia
- Hypokalaemia
- Disequilibration syndrome (cerebral oedema)
- Dialysis-related amyloidosis (β_2-microglobulin accumulation causing peripheral neuropathy, etc.)

Side-effects of post-transplant immunosuppressive drug therapy

- High-dose corticosteroids [p82]
  - Cushingoid facies (moon face, plethora, acne, hirsute)
  - Thin skin
  - Bruising
  - Abdominal obesity
  - Purple striae
  - Muscle wasting in limbs
- Ciclosporin
  - Gingival hypertrophy
  - Warty skin lesions
  - Hypertrichosis (werewolf syndrome)

NOTES

The GALS screen is a different type of examination. Rather than following a conventional sequence (e.g. look, feel, move...) you jump between these in the interests of efficiency & speed. This is because the GALS examination was designed as a rapid screening tool to be used when clerking patients admitted to hospital (taking 1–2 min). The downside is that it is difficult to remember, so practice it well. The sequence is really Gait – General inspection – Spine – Arms – Legs, but GGISAL isn't quite as snappy as GALS!

	Action / Examine for	ΔΔ / Potential findings / Extra information

Introduction	• Wash / gel hands
	• Introduce yourself, confirm pt, explain examination & gain consent
	• Expose pt (top off, shorts only, no socks / shoes)
	• Ask the 3 'GALS questions'
	  1. *"Do you have any pain or stiffness in your muscles, joints or back?"*
	  2. *"Can you dress yourself completely without any difficulty?"*
	  3. *"Are you able to walk up and down stairs without difficulty?"*
		→ Consider chaperone

Gait	• Ask pt to walk across room, turn and walk back
	• Consider features of gait
	  ○ Symmetry
	  ○ Smoothness
	  ○ Normal heel strike then toe-off
	  ○ Normal step height
		→ [↩]

Patient standing		

General inspection — **From behind**	• Look (head to toe)
	  ○ Shoulder muscle bulk & symmetry
	  ○ Spinal alignment
	  ○ Iliac crest alignment
	  ○ Gluteal muscle bulk & symmetry
	  ○ Popliteal swelling
	  ○ Calf muscle bulk & symmetry
	  ○ Hindfoot abnormality / deformity
		→ S-shaped spine = scoliosis
		→ Pelvic tilt can indicate hip abductor weakness
		→ Baker's cyst, popliteal aneurysm (pulsatile – feel to check if unsure)

General inspection — **From the side**	• Look (head to toe)
	  ○ Normal cervical lordosis
	  ○ Normal thoracic kyphosis
	  ○ Normal lumbar lordosis
	  ○ Knee flexion / hyperextension	

General inspection — **From in front**	• Look (head to toe)
	  ○ Shoulder muscle bulk & symmetry
	  ○ Elbow extension
	  ○ Quadriceps muscle bulk & symmetry
	  ○ Knee swelling / deformity
	  ○ Foot arches
	  ○ Midfoot & forefoot abnormality / deformity
		→ High arches = pes cavus, flat feet = pes planus

GALS SCREEN

GALS SCREEN

Section	Region	Assessment	Notes

Spine	**Cervical spine**	• Move
		  ○ Lateral flexion: *"Try to touch your ear to each shoulder"*
		  ○ Flexion: *"Put your chin down onto your chest"*
		  ○ Extension: *"Put your head back as far as possible"*
		  ○ Rotation: *"Look over each shoulder"*
			→ If limited, pt may cheat by bringing shoulder up towards ear

	Lumbar spine	• Move
		  ○ Flexion: *"Try to touch your toes"*
		  ○ Observe degree of hip & lumbar spine flexion
		  ○ Confirm lumbar spine flexion by asking pt to repeat the manoeuvre with your index & middle fingers on the spinous processes of 2 adjacent lumbar vertebrae
			→ Your fingers will separate with lumbar flexion

Arms	**Shoulders & elbows**	• Move
		  ○ Shoulder ABduction / external rotation & elbow flexion:
		    "Put both hands behind your head"	

	Hands	• Look
		  ○ Swelling / deformity / muscle wasting
		• Feel
		  ○ Squeeze MCP joints to check for tenderness
		• Move
		  ○ Pronation / supination
		  ○ Power grip: *"Squeeze my fingers tightly"*
		  ○ Fine pincer grip: *"Touch your thumb to each finger in turn"*
			→ Sign of synovitis and possible inflammatory arthropathy

Legs
Lying flat with 1 pillow
	Hips & knees	• Feel
		  ○ Patellar tap
		    ■ Leg straight, compress suprapatellar bursa with one hand
		    ■ Attempt to 'bounce' patella with other hand
		• Move
		  ○ Active hip & knee flexion: *"Bring your knee up towards your chin"*
		  ○ Passive hip internal rotation (hip at 90°, knee at 90°, hold knee & ankle, gently move foot away from other leg)
			→ Painful / limited early in hip OA

	Feet	• Look
		  ○ Swelling / deformity / callus formation
		• Feel
		  ○ Squeeze MTP joints to check for tenderness
			→ Abnormal pattern of calluses may be caused by gait abnormality
			→ Sign of synovitis and possible inflammatory arthropathy

	Conclusion	○ Wash / gel hands, thank pt & allow to re-dress ○ If areas of concern: *"I would like to assess [joint] in more detail"*	→ GALS is a screening test

Gait abnormalities

	Features	Causes
Antalgic	• Less time spent on painful limb (a limp)	• Pathology of hip / knee / ankle

Trendelenburg	• Waddling gait	• Hip ABductor weakness
		  ○ Nerve lesion
		  ○ Root lesion
		  ○ Muscular dystrophy
		  ○ Myopathy
		  ○ Polio
		• # NOF
		• DDH
		• SUFE

Parkinsonian
[p76]
	• Hesitation
	• Shuffling
	• Loss of arm swing
	• Hurried steps – 'marche à petit pas'
	• Festination (speeding up inadvertently)
	• Retropulsion (falling backwards as feet rush ahead)
		• Parkinsonism
		  ○ Parkinson's disease
		  ○ Drug-induced
		  ○ Parkinson-plus syndrome
		• Atherosclerotic pseudoparkinsonism

Sensory ataxic	• Broad-based
	• Looking at feet
		• Sensory peripheral neuropathy
		• Dorsal column loss
		  ○ MS
		  ○ SCDC
		  ○ Tabes dorsalis

Cerebellar [p80]	• Broad-based • High-stepping • Looking carefully ahead	• Cerebellar lesion (usually vermis)

Hemiplegic	• Foot plantarflexed and knee extended
	• Leg must be abducted and swung in a lateral arc
	• Arm may also be held in UMN posture
		• UMN lesion
		  ○ Stroke
		  ○ Tumour
		  ○ MS

Foot-drop	• High-stepping to allow toes to clear ground	• Common peroneal nerve palsy • Sciatic nerve palsy • L4 / L5 root lesion • MND • Peripheral motor neuropathy (e.g. alcoholic)

GALS SCREEN NOTES

Acute monoarthritis / oligoarthritis

- Initial investigations
  - XR
  - Inflammatory markers (FBC for WCC & differential, CRP, ESR)
  - Blood cultures if pyrexial
  - Consider joint aspiration (send synovial fluid for microscopy for crystals, gram stain & culture)
- Consider ΔΔ – **GRASP** (see table below)
- An acutely inflamed joint is septic until proven otherwise
- If pt systemically unwell aspirate joint, take blood cultures then start empirical antibiotics
- Consider haemarthrosis in ΔΔ particularly if history of coagulopathy (e.g. haemophilia)

	Typical age	Typical gender	Typical joint involvement	Other information	Specific Ix
Gout	Middle age to elderly	Male > Female	1st MTPJ > ankle > knee > upper limb	• Polyarticular in 10%	• Serum urate
Reactive Arthritis	Young	Male > Female	Lower limb large joint (usually > 1 joint involved)	• Associated with GI & GUM infections • Take GI, GU & sexual history • Look for rash, balanitis, conjunctivitis	• Stool sample • STD swabs
Septic Joint	Any age	Male or Female	Any joint	• Usually staphylococcus in adults • Consider gonococcus in young adults	
Pseudogout	Middle age to elderly	Male or Female	Knee or wrist	• Can mimic gout or sepsis	• Chondrocalcinosis on XR

NOTES

A note on musculoskeletal examination sequence

A commonly used musculoskeletal examination sequence is look, feel, move, special tests, function, distal neurovascular integrity. Alternatively, function (e.g. gait) can be assessed at the start to identify any abnormality and tailor the rest of the examination to focus on this.

However, in the case of several joint examinations (the lower limb ones in particular) this sequence is disrupted by the need to change patient position (e.g. from supine to standing). To complete an efficient examination and avoid repeatedly standing the patient up then lying them back down, it is necessary to modify the sequence.

	Action / Examine for	ΔΔ / Potential findings / Extra information

Introduction	• Wash / gel hands
	• Introduce yourself, confirm pt, explain examination & gain consent
	• Expose & position pt (down to pants or shorts, supine with 1 pillow)
	  "Which hip is sore? Where is it sore?"
	  "I would like to compare the affected hip with the unaffected one"
		→ Consider chaperone
		
		→ Examiner may ask you to proceed with examination of just one hip

Look	• Age and general physical condition of pt (BMI, frailty)
	• Mobility aids
	• Hips
	  ○ Symmetry (compare sides)
	  ○ Muscle wasting
	  ○ Scars
	  ○ Redness
	  ○ Swelling
	  ○ Fixed flexion (look from the side)
	  ○ External rotation of leg (look at foot)
	• Measure leg length with tape measure
	  ○ True: ASIS to medial maleolus
	  ○ Apparent: Umbilicus to medial maleolus
		→ Crutches, walking stick, wheelchair, etc.
		
		→ Arthroscopy, arthroplasty, DHS
		→ Inflammation
		→ Inflammation, effusion
		→ OA, other hip pathology
		→ # NOF (acute or malunion)
		   [↔]

Feel	• Temperature – use back of hand and compare sides
	  ○ Anterior hip joint
	  ○ Over greater trochanter (lateral thigh)
	  "Tell me if I cause you any discomfort"
	• Hip in neutral position
	  ○ Palpate ASIS
	  ○ Palpate anterior joint line (deep)
	  ○ Palpate greater trochanter (lateral)
		→ Warmth indicates inflammation
		
		→ Feel for tenderness, bony abnormality (e.g. osteophytes)
		→ Trochanteric bursitis (trauma, OA)

Move	• Assess ROM & pain on movement
	• Active movement
	  ○ Flexion – *"Bring your knee right up to your chest"*
	  ○ ABduction / ADduction (cross one straight leg over the other)
	  ○ Conjugate hip movement – *"Lift your foot off the bed and make circles with it in the air"*
		→ Normal 120° – you could assess passive flexion beyond this
		
		→ Useful test of general hip function

HIP

Move – cont'd	• Passive movement – "*Tell me if this causes any discomfort*"	→ Watch pt's face for evidence of discomfort
	○ Flex both hip & knee to 90°, hold ankle & knee	
	■ Internal rotation (move foot *away* from other leg)	→ Normal 40° (often limited & painful in hip OA)
	■ External rotation (move foot *towards* other leg)	→ Normal 30°
	○ Legs straight, stabilise pelvis by laying forearm across ASISs	
	■ ABduction	→ Normal 45° (first to be limited by OA)
	■ ADduction	→ Normal 30°
	○ If possible, roll pt onto side	→ Normal 20°, may not be able to roll onto bad hip
	■ Extension	
Special tests	• Thomas test [↪ *Fig. 1*]	→ Fixed flexion deformity
	○ Place left hand in hollow of pt's lumbar spine	○ OA
	○ Passively flex right hip with right hand up to limit of ROM	○ Other hip pathology
	○ With left hand feel that the lumbar lordosis has flattened	
	○ Positive test: left thigh rises up	→ Fixed flexion deformity of left hip
	○ Repeat on the other side	

Patient standing

Look (again)	• Inspect from the front, sides & back	
	○ Deformity / muscle wasting may become more obvious	
Function	• Ask pt to walk across room and back	[p24]
	• Consider features of gait	→ Antalgic gait (limp), wobbling Trendelenburg gait (see below)
	○ Symmetry & smoothness	
	○ Normal heel strike, toe off & step height	
Special tests (again)	• Trendelenburg test [↪ *Fig. 2, Fig. 3*]	→ ABductor instability
	○ Sit on a chair in front of pt	○ Pain (e.g. OA)
	○ Place your hands on their iliac crests with your thumbs over ASISs	○ Weakness (e.g. nerve root lesion)
	○ "*Put your hands on my shoulders or hold my arms & support yourself*"	○ DDH
	○ Ask pt to stand on one leg at a time – the 'good leg' first	○ SUFE
	○ Normal: pelvis tilts upwards on unsupported side	
	○ Positive test: pelvis tilts downwards on unsupported side & trunk leans	→ When walking this results in the wobbling Trendelenburg gait
	in opposite direction to maintain balance	
Neurovascular Integrity	• Sensation on dorsal foot & sole of foot	
	• Dorsalis pedis & posterior tibial pulses, CRT (hallux)	
Conclusion	• Wash / gel hands, thank pt & allow to re-dress	→ Particularly the joint above & below
	• If not done: "*I would like to examine the other hip*"	→ Pattern of joint involvement can aid diagnosis
	• "*I would like to examine the knee and lumbar spine, then go on to*	→ Weightbearing X-rays can be useful
	perform a full musculoskeletal assessment"	
	• Investigations: X-rays, CT hip, joint aspiration	

HIP

Leg length shortening

- Apparent – due to pelvic tilting
  - Fixed flexion deformity of hip
  - Fixed ADduction deformity of hip (especially OA)
- True – due to joint or bony abnormality
  - Pathology distal to trochanters
    - Previous # femur
    - Previous # tibia
    - Growth disturbance (polio, epiphyseal trauma)
  - Pathology proximal to trochanters
    - # NOF
    - OA
    - Hip dislocation

Total hip replacement

- Indications
  - OA
  - Less commonly RA / DDH / seronegative arthropathy
  - Displaced intracapsular NOF # in young pt [see below]
- Complications
  - Perioperative (anaesthetic-related, haemorrhage, infection)
  - Acute dislocation
  - Chronic infection
- Contraindications
  - Mild disease
  - Doubt as to origin of hip pain
  - Morbid obesity

Neck of femur

- Usually elderly, osteoporotic pt following low-velocity fall onto hip
- Blood supply to the femoral head
  1. Cervical arteries running in the joint capsule retinaculum (*main supply*)
  2. Intramedullary vessels in the femoral neck
  3. Vessels of the ligamentum teres (negligible contribution, often non-existent)
- Displaced intracapsular #
  - Inevitable interruption of intramedullary vessels and likely disruption of cervical arteries
  - High risk of avascular necrosis (AVN) of femoral head
  - Usually treated by hip replacement
    - hemi-arthroplasty in older pts
    - total hip replacement in younger pts likely to be more active post-op
- Undisplaced intracapsular #
  - Inevitable interruption of intramedullary vessels, possible disruption to cervical arteries
  - Moderate risk of AVN
  - Usually pinned in the hope that AVN will not develop (~30% risk)
- Intertrochanteric or subtrochanteric extracapsular #
  - Little interruption to blood supply of femoral head
  - Low risk of AVN
  - Usually stabilised and reduced using dynamic hip screw

Hip flexors
- Psoas
- Iliacus
- Tensor fasciae latae
- Sartorius
- Pectineus
- ADductor longus
- ADductor brevis
- Rectus femoris (one of the quadriceps)

Hip extensors
- Gluteus maximus
- Hamstrings

Hip ABductors
- Gluteus medius & minimus

Hip ADductors
- ADductor magnus, longus & brevis

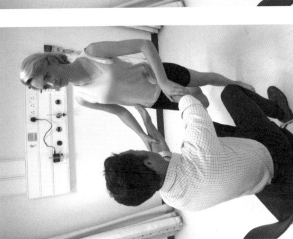
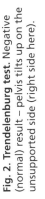
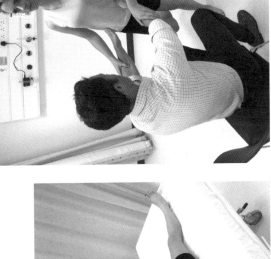

Fig. 3. Trendelenburg test. Positive (abnormal) result due to hip ABductor instability – pelvis drops down on the unsupported (right) side & trunk leans to the opposite (left) side to keep balance.

Fig. 2. Trendelenburg test. Negative (normal) result – pelvis tilts up on the unsupported side (right side here).

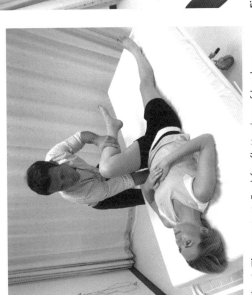

Fig. 1. Thomas test. Feel for flattening of lumbar lordosis & look for opposite thigh rising up due to a fixed flexion deformity of that hip. It is also important to watch the patient's face to ensure you don't cause pain.

HIP NOTES

KNEE

	Action / Examine for	ΔΔ / Potential findings / Extra information
Introduction	• Wash / gel hands • Introduce yourself, confirm pt, explain examination & gain consent • Expose & position pt (down to pants / shorts, lie flat with 1 pillow) • *"Which knee is sore? Where is it sore?"* • *"I would like to compare the affected knee with the unaffected one"*	→ Consider chaperone → Examiner may ask you to proceed with examination of just one knee

Look	• Age and general physical condition of pt (BMI, frailty)
	• Mobility aids
	• Knees
	  ○ Symmetry (compare sides)
	  ○ Muscle wasting
	  ○ Scars
	  ○ Redness
	  ○ Swelling
	  ○ Fixed flexion (look from the side)
	  ○ Measure thigh circumference 10 cm above patella, compare sides
		→ Walking stick, crutch, wheelchair, etc.
		→ Deformity – valgus & [handwritten]
		→ Arthroscopy (small), knee replacement (large, anterior crossing joint)
		→ Inflammation
		→ Inflammation, effusion, Baker's cyst
		→ OA, other knee pathology
		→ Hamstring / quadriceps wasting

Feel	• Temperature – use back of hand & compare sides
	  ○ Superior to patella
	  ○ Medial & lateral joint lines
	• *"Tell me if I cause you any discomfort"*
	• With knee flexed to 90°
	  ○ Palpate medial & lateral joint lines
	  ○ Palpate patellar tendon insertion (tibial tuberosity)
	• With leg straight
	  ○ Palpate patellar border & quadriceps tendon
	  ○ Palpate behind knee for swelling
	• Patellar tap
	  ○ Leg straight, compress suprapatellar bursa with one hand
	  ○ Attempt to 'bounce' patella with other hand
	• Sweep test
	  ○ Leg straight, run hand up medial side of knee 2–3 times
	  ○ Immediately run hand *down* lateral side of knee
	  ○ Watch for 'bulge' of fluid in medial compartment
		→ Warmth = sign of inflammation
		→ Feel for tenderness, bony abnormality (e.g. osteophytes)
		→ Baker's cyst, popliteal aneurysm
		→ Large knee effusion
		→ Small knee effusion (more sensitive than patellar tap)

Move	• Assess ROM & pain on movement
	• Active movement
	  ○ Flexion – *"Bring your heel right into your bottom"*
	  ○ Extension – *"Straighten your leg out again"*
	  ○ Hyperextension – *"Push the back of your knee into the bed"*
	  ○ Straight leg raise – *"Keep your leg straight, raise your heel off the bed"*
	• Passive movement – *"Tell me if this causes any discomfort"*
	  ○ Flexion & extension with hand on top of patella
		→ Normal 140°
		→ 10° hyperextension normal
		→ Integrity of extensor mechanism
		→ Watch pt's face for evidence of discomfort
		→ Feel for crepitus

Special tests (perform as one sequence)	• Anterior & posterior drawer tests [⇨ *Fig. 4 & Fig. 5*]
	  ○ Flex knee to 90°
	  ○ Look from side for posterior sag
	  ○ Sit on pt's foot
	  ○ Grab behind knee with both hands, thumbs on tibial tuberosity
	  ○ Stabilizing lower tibia with your forearms
	  ○ Anterior drawer: attempt to pull tibia forwards on the femur
	  ○ Posterior drawer: now attempt to push tibia backwards on the femur
		→ ACL (anterior drawer) & PCL (posterior drawer) integrity
		→ PCL integrity
		→ Feel hamstrings & ensure relaxed
		
		→ Should be little movement & firm end-point with intact ACL
		→ Should be little movement & firm end-point with intact PCL

	• McMurray's test [⇨ *Fig. 6*]
	  ○ Flex knee and hip to 90°
	  ○ Grasp sole of foot with one hand
	  ○ Grasp knee with other hand, thumb feeling down one joint line and index finger feeling down the other
	  ○ Straighten knee with foot held in external then internal rotation
	  ○ Feel for 'click' and look for pt discomfort
		→ Meniscal tear

	• Collateral ligament stress test [⇨ *Fig. 7*]
	  ○ Flex knee to 15°
	  ○ Grasp foot with one hand, support knee with the other
	  ○ Stress each side of the knee in turn, feeling for laxity
		→ MCL / LCL weakness

	• Patellar apprehension test [⇨ *Fig. 8*]
	  ○ Leg straight
	  ○ Apply lateral force to patella, begin to flex knee, watching face
	  ○ If pt 'apprehensive' and doesn't allow this = positive test
		→ Previous patellar dislocation

Patient standing		

Look (again)	• Inspect from the front, sides & back
	  ○ Deformity, muscle wasting may be more obvious than when supine
	  ○ Varus deformity (bow-legged)
	  ○ Valgus deformity (knock-kneed)
		→ Particularly varus / valgus deformity
		→ OA, rickets (historically)
		→ OA, RA

Function	• Ask pt to walk across room and back
	• Consider features of gait
	  ○ Symmetry & smoothness
	  ○ Normal heel strike, toe-off & step height
		→ [p24]
		→ Antalgic gait (limp)

Neurovascular Integrity	• Sensation on dorsal foot & sole of foot • Dorsalis pedis & posterior tibial pulses, CRT in hallux	
Conclusion	• Wash / gel hands, thank pt & allow to re-dress • If not done: " *I would like to examine the other knee* " • " *I would like to examine the hip and ankle, then go on to perform a full musculoskeletal assessment* " • Investigations: X-rays, MRI, aspiration of effusion	→ Joint above & below → Pattern of joint involvement can aid diagnosis → Weightbearing X-rays can be useful

KNEE

Hamstring muscles (knee flexors)
- Semitendinosis
- Semimembranosus
- Biceps femoris

Quadriceps muscles (knee extensors)
- Rectus femoris
- Vastus lateralis
- Vastus intermedius
- Vastus medialis

Knee osteoarthritis
- Very common
- May affect
  - Medial compartment
  - Lateral compartment
  - Patellofemoral compartment
  - All 3 (tricompartmental OA)
- Treatment
  - Conservative
    - Analgesia
    - Physiotherapy
    - Walking aids
  - Operative
    - Total knee replacement

Meniscal injuries
- Relatively common
- Young pt – likely purely traumatic tear of medial meniscus
- Older pt – increased chance of degenerative tear of lateral meniscus
- Loose meniscal fragment may enter joint space, causing locking (inability to extend knee)

Common peroneal nerve
- Anatomy
  - Descends obliquely along lateral side of popliteal fossa
  - Winds around fibular neck
  - Superficial branch innervates muscles of lateral leg compartment (foot eversion)
  - Deep branch innervates muscles of the anterior leg compartment (foot dorsiflexion)
  - Sensory supply to lateral leg and dorsum of foot
- Injury
  - Trauma to lateral leg at the level of fibular head
  - Classicallly being hit by a car bumper
  - Most significant consequence is loss of foot dorsiflexion, leading to foot drop
  - Results in high-stepping gait [p24]

KNEE NOTES

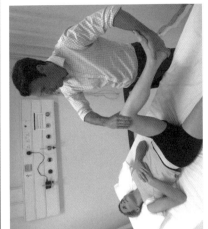

Fig. 6. McMurray's test. Looks for evidence of meniscal tear. Perform with foot held in external, then internal rotation.

NOTES

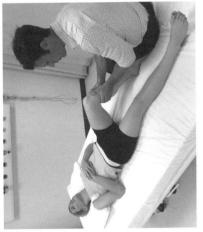

Fig. 5. Posterior drawer test. Push the tibia backwards on the femur to assess PCL integrity.

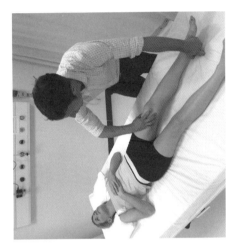

Fig. 8. Patellar apprehension test. Previous patellar dislocation.

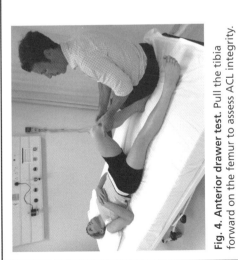

Fig. 4. Anterior drawer test. Pull the tibia forward on the femur to assess ACL integrity.

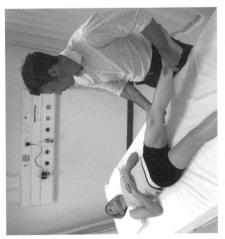

Fig. 7. Collateral ligament stress test. Here the MCL is being assessed for laxity. Swap hands to assess the LCL.

	Action / Examine for	ΔΔ / Potential findings / Extra information
Introduction	• Wash / gel hands • Introduce yourself, confirm pt, explain examination & gain consent • Expose & position pt (bare from knees down, supine at 45° with feet hanging over the end of the examination couch) • *"Which foot is sore? Where is it sore?"* • *"I would like to compare the affected foot with the unaffected one"*	→ Examiner may ask you to examine just one foot / ankle

Look	• Age & general physical condition of pt (BMI, frailty)
	• Mobility aids
	• Footwear
	  ○ Orthotics / insoles
	  ○ Asymmetrical wear on soles
	• Ankles & dorsal surface of feet
	  ○ Symmetry (compare sides)
	  ○ Deformity
	  ○ Skin changes
	  ○ Redness / swelling
	  ○ Scars
	  ○ Muscle wasting
	  ○ Nails
	• Between toes
	• Plantar surface of feet (from below)
	  ○ Normal skin thickening under 1st MTP joint & heel
	  ○ Abnormal callus formation elsewhere
	• Posterior heel & Achilles tendon
	  ○ Redness / swelling
		→ Crutches, walking stick, wheelchair, etc.
		
		→ Due to abnormal gait or pressure loading
		
		→ Missing toes, hallux valgus +/− bunion, hammer/mallet/claw toe, CMT
		→ Atrophy, ulceration, discolouration, hair loss, psoriasis
		→ Inflammation
		
		→ Onycholysis (psoriasis), atrophic change (diabetes, arterial insufficiency)
		→ Infection, hidden ulcers
		→ Due to normal pressure loading
		→ Due to deformity / gait abnormality & abnormal pressure loading

Feel	• Temperature – use back of hand & compare sides
	  ○ Over MTP joints, dorsal midfoot, medial / anterior / lateral ankle
	• *"Tell me if I cause you any discomfort"*
	  ○ Squeeze across individual toe joints
	  ○ Squeeze across MTP joints
	  ○ Squeeze across midfoot
	  ○ Palpate subtalar joint medially & laterally just distal to malleoli
	  ○ Palpate medial malleolus
	  ○ Palpate anterior ankle joint line
	  ○ Palpate lateral malleolus
	  ○ Palpate Achilles tendon
		→ Hot (inflammation) or cold (arterial insufficiency)
		
		→ Thickening, tenderness

Move	• Assess ROM and pain on movement
	• Active movement
	  ○ Inversion / eversion
	    ■ Stabilise above ankle with one hand
	    ■ Put your other index finger in space just medial / lateral to foot
	    ■ *"Move your foot to try and touch my finger"*
		→ Normal 30° / 20°

FOOT AND ANKLE

Move – contd	○ Great toe dorsiflexion / plantarflexion
	   ■ Stabilise midfoot with your hand to eliminate ankle movement
	   ■ *"Pull your big toe up towards your nose"*
	   ■ *"Curl your big toe down as much as possible"*
	○ Ankle dorsiflexion / plantarflexion
		→ Normal 20° / 40°

	• Passive movement – *"Tell me if I cause you any discomfort"*
	○ Assess any joint that is abnormal
	  (red, hot, swollen, deformed, reduced ROM on active movement)
	○ Midtarsal joint movement (only assessed passively)
	   ■ Stabilise directly over ankle joint with your left hand
	   ■ Grasp forefoot with your right hand
	   ■ Apply twisting motion between your hands
	○ Subtalar joint movement (only assessed passively)
	   ■ Stabilise above ankle joint with your left hand
	   ■ Grasp heel with your right hand
	   ■ Invert / evert the foot
		→ Watch pt's face for evidence of discomfort

Special tests	• Simmonds' test [⇨ *Fig. 9*] ○ Pt prone with feet hanging off end of examination couch ○ Squeeze the belly of the calf and look for ankle plantarflexion ○ Absence of plantarflexion suggests Achilles tendon rupture	→ Achilles tendon integrity
Patient standing		
Look (again)	• Heel alignment (look from behind) • Medial arches • If flat feet ask to stand on tip toes & observe whether correction occurs	→ Varus or valgus deformity → Pes cavus (high arched feet), pes planus (flat feet) → Differentiate between flexible & fixed flat feet
Function	• Ask pt to walk across room and back and consider features of gait ○ Symmetry & smoothness ○ Normal heel strike ○ Normal toe-off ○ Normal step height	→ [p 24] → Pt may avoid heel strike if hindfoot painful → Pt may avoid toe push-off if forefoot painful → High stepping gait in foot drop
Neurovascular integrity	• Sensation on plantar surfaces of hallux, MTP joints & heel • Sensory level on legs if peripheral neuropathy suspected ○ Tap cotton wool up antero-medial leg starting at tip of hallux ○ Ask pt to tell you when they feel sensation *change* ○ Repeat on other leg • Ankle jerk reflexes • Dorsalis pedis & posterior tibial pulses, CRT in hallux • ABPI if arterial insufficiency suspected	→ [p 62] → 'Glove and stocking' sensory loss (e.g. diabetic neuropathy) → May be reduced / absent in peripheral neuropathy
Conclusion	• Wash / gel hands, thank pt & allow to re-dress • If not done: *"I would like to examine the other foot and ankle"* • *"I would like to examine the knees and hips, then go on to complete a full musculoskeletal assessment"* • More detailed neurological or vascular assessments if deficit identified • Investigations: X-rays, MRI, joint aspiration	

FOOT AND ANKLE

Diabetic foot features
- Peripheral neuropathy
  - Particularly loss of ankle jerks & vibration sense on examination
  - Accidental injury & tissue damage
  - Charcot joints (see below)
- Autonomic neuropathy
  - Reduced sweating
  - Dry, cracked skin predisposing to infection
- Arterial insufficiency
  - Large vessel disease
  - Small vessel disease
- All of the above contribute to ulcer formation

Charcot joints
- Also known as neuropathic joints
- Most common cause is diabetic neuropathy
- Other causes
  - Tabes dorsalis (syphilis – historically a major cause)
  - Cerebral palsy
  - Spinal cord injury
  - Syringomyelia
- Loss of sensation & proprioception to weight-bearing joint results in repeated trauma
- Joint becomes severely damaged and disrupted over time leading to deformity
- Often still painful despite the neuropathy
- Often associated ulceration and/or infection

Charcot–Marie–Tooth disease
- Group of inherited disorders of the peripheral nervous system
- Mixed motor & sensory peripheral neuropathy
- Progressive loss of muscle tissue and loss of touch sensation
- Foot drop usually present
- Hammer / claw toes
- Muscle wasting in lower legs leads to 'inverted champagne bottle' appearance
- High arched feet (pes cavus) or flat arched feet (pes planus)

FOOT AND ANKLE NOTES

Ankle joints*

- True ankle joint
  - Talocrural joint
  - Articulation between distal tibia / fibula and talus
  - Hinge joint
  - Dorsiflexion / plantarflexion
- Subtalar joint
  - Talocalcaneal joint
  - Articulation between talus & calcaneus
  - Condyloid joint
  - Inversion / eversion

*This is a simplification – in reality the biomechanics of the ankle joint are highly complex.

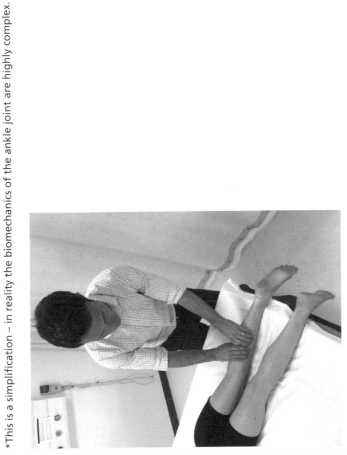

Fig. 9. Simmonds test. Achilles tendon integrity. Normally you will see foot plantarflexion when you squeeze belly of calf.

	Action / Examine for	ΔΔ / Potential findings / Extra information
Introduction	• Wash / gel hands • Introduce yourself, confirm pt, explain examination & gain consent • Expose & position pt (top off, standing) • *"Which shoulder is sore? Can you point to where it is painful?"* • *"I would like to compare the affected shoulder with the unaffected one"*	→ Consider chaperone → Examiner may ask you to proceed with examination of just one shoulder

Look	• Age and general condition of pt (BMI, frailty)
	• Disability aids
	• From front, sides & back
	  ○ Symmetry (compare sides)
	  ○ Muscle wasting
	  ○ Scars
	  ○ Redness / swelling
	  ○ Deformity including winged scapula
	• Check axillae for obvious abnormality
		→ Age important in determining likely cause of shoulder pain [↔]
		
		→ Deltoid – axillary nerve palsy
		→ Arthroscopy, shoulder replacement
		→ Inflammation
		→ Long thoracic nerve palsy

Feel	• Temperature
	  ○ Use back of hand & compare sides
	  ○ Anterior & posterior shoulder
	• *"Tell me if I cause you any discomfort"*
	  ○ Palpate sternoclavicular joint, clavicle & AC joint
	  ○ Palpate anterior joint, long head of biceps & posterior joint
	  ○ Palpate borders of scapula
		→ Warmth indicates inflammation
		
		→ Feel for tenderness, bony abnormality (e.g. osteophytes)

Move	• Assess ROM and pain on movement
	• Active movement
	  ○ Looking from the side
	    ■ Flexion
	    ■ Extension
	  ○ Looking from behind
	    ■ ABduction
	    ■ Slow ABduction as you stabilise tip of scapula
	    ■ Internal rotation (reach up middle of back)
	  ○ Looking from in front
	    ■ External rotation (elbows flexed to 90° and tucked into sides)
	• Passive movement – *"Tell me if I cause you any discomfort"*
	  ○ All above movements with hand on top of shoulder
	  ○ Slow ABduction to detect painful arc
		→ Both shoulders at once (unless you have been told to examine one only)
		
		→ Normal 180°
		→ Normal 60°
		
		→ Normal 180°
		→ Ratio of true gleno-humeral to scapular movement (normally 2:1)
		→ Normal 90°
		
		→ Normal 70–90°, particularly limited with frozen shoulder [↔]
		→ Watch pt's face for evidence of discomfort
		→ Feel for crepitus
		→ Impingement syndrome [↔]

SHOULDER

Special tests (divided by the pathology which they test for)	• Shoulder instability – shoulder apprehension test [↪ *Fig. 10*]
	  ○ Best done with pt supine
	  ○ ABduct shoulder 90°, flex elbow 90°, externally rotate shoulder
	  ○ Stabilise pt's elbow with one hand
	  ○ Force further external rotation with other hand
	  ○ 'Apprehensive' reaction to this = positive test
		→ Young pts, usually previous dislocation
		→ All other tests conducted standing
		→ Forearm nearing horizontal

	• Impingement syndrome – Hawkin's test [↪ *Fig. 11*]
	  ○ Flex shoulder 90°, flex elbow 90°, internally rotate shoulder
	  ○ Stabilise pt's elbow with one hand
	  ○ Force further internal rotation with other hand
	  ○ Pain in shoulder = positive test
		→ Push downwards on pt's hand
		
		→ Middle-aged pts
		→ Forearm pointing downwards
		
		→ Push downwards on pt's hand

	• Rotator cuff injury (supraspinatus) – Jobe's test [↪ *Fig. 12*]
	  ○ 'Gladiator' position
	  ○ Straight arm ABducted to 90°, thumb pointed at floor
	  ○ *"Keep your arm up, don't let me push it down"*
	  ○ Force shoulder ADduction against resistance from pt
	  ○ Pain / difficulty = positive test
		→ Older pts
		
		→ Push downwards on pt's hand
		→ May also be painful if impingement present

	• Rotator cuff injury (subscapularis) – Gerber's lift-off test [↪ *Fig. 13*]
	  ○ Hand behind back, dorsum resting against mid-lumbar spine
	  ○ Stand behind pt
	  ○ Apply light pressure to pt's outward-facing palm
	  ○ *"Push your hand straight backwards, off your back"*
	  ○ Pain / difficulty = positive test
		→ Older pts

	• Rotator cuff injury (teres minor & infraspinatus) – resisted external rotation [↪ *Fig. 14*]
	  ○ Arms by sides, elbows flexed to 90°
	  ○ Ask to externally rotate shoulders whilst you oppose them
	  ○ Pain / difficulty = positive test
		→ Older pts
		
		→ Apply 'inwards' pressure to hands

Function	• Both hands behind head • Both hands up to mouth • Both hands down to bottom	→ Washing hair, dressing → Eating → Cleaning after toilet

Neurovascular integrity	• Sensation
	  ○ Axillary: Regimental badge area
	  ○ Median: Lateral aspect of index finger
	  ○ Ulnar: Medial aspect of little finger
	  ○ Radial: Dorsal 1st interosseous space
	  ○ Radial pulse & CRT in finger
		→ Anterior shoulder dislocation
		
		} [p57]

Conclusion	• Wash / gel hands; thank pt & allow them to re-dress • If not done: *"I would like to examine the other shoulder"* • *"I would like to examine the elbow and cervical spine, and then go on to examine the rest of the musculoskeletal system"* • Investigations: X-rays (AP & modified axillary views), MRI, joint aspiration	→ Joint above and below → Pattern of joint involvement can aid diagnosis

SHOULDER

Common shoulder pathology

1. Instability
   - Usually young pt
   - Previous dislocation(s)
   - Shoulder apprehension test
2. Impingement syndrome
   - Usually middle-aged pt
   - Hawkin's test
3. Rotator cuff tear
   - Usually older pt – 'grey hair cuff tear'
   - Test components of rotator cuff
     - Supraspinatus
       – Anterosuperior cuff
       – Jobe's test
     - Subscapularis
       – Anteroinferior cuff
       – Gerber's lift-off test
     - Teres minor & infraspinatus
       – Posterior cuff
       – Resisted external shoulder rotation

Complications of anterior dislocation of shoulder (95% of dislocations are anterior)

- Axillary nerve damage
- Brachial plexus / other nerve damage
- Axillary artery damage
- Associated fracture (30% of cases)
  - Humeral head
  - Clavicle
  - Acromion
- Recurrent shoulder dislocation
- Anatomical lesion
  - Bankart
  - Hill–Sachs
- Rotator cuff injury

Impingement syndrome

- Also known as painful arc syndrome
- Underlying pathology is supraspinatus tendonitis
- Painful arc
  - Classical sign of supraspinatus tendonitis
  - Pain during shoulder ABduction between 60° and 120°
  - Due to 'impingement' of the underside of the acromion on the inflamed tendon
- Positive Hawkin's test
  - Arm flexed to 90°
  - Elbow flexed to 90°
  - Shoulder internally rotated, pushing supraspinatus tendon up against acromion
  - Forcing further internal rotation causes pain if tendon is inflamed
  - (Note Jobe's test for supraspinatus weakness/tear may also cause pain)

Frozen shoulder

- Adhesive capsulitis of glenohumeral joint
- Most commonly affects ages 40–65
- Can occur
  - Spontaneously
  - Following rotor cuff injury
  - Following immobility (e.g. stroke)
- Diabetes & thyroid disease are risk factors
- Phases
  - Freezing phase
    - gradual onset of shoulder pain and stiffness
    - 2–9 months
  - Frozen phase
    - pain subsides but stiffness remains
    - external rotation usually very limited
    - 4–12 months
  - Thawing phase
    - gradual return of movement
    - recovery may be incomplete
    - 1–3 years

NOTES

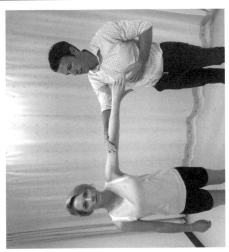

Fig. 12. Jobe's test. Supraspinatous pathology.

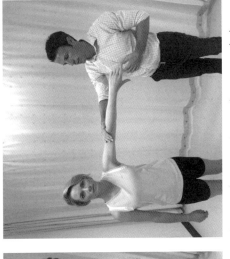

Fig. 11. Hawkins test. Impingement syndrome.

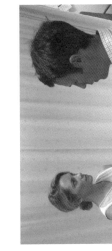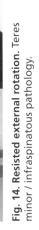

Fig. 14. Resisted external rotation. Teres minor / infraspinatous pathology.

Fig. 10. Shoulder apprehension test. Shoulder instability (usually previous dislocation).

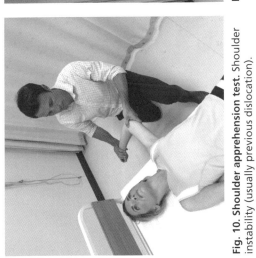

Fig. 13. Gerber's lift-off test. Subscapularis pathology.

	Action / Examine for	ΔΔ / Potential findings / Extra information
Introduction	• Wash / gel hands • Introduce yourself, confirm pt, explain examination & gain consent • Expose & position pt (bare below shoulders, standing, arms by sides, palms facing forward) • *"Which elbow is sore? Where is it sore?"* • *"I would like to compare the affected elbow with the unaffected one"*	→ Ideally in a t-shirt or vest rather than rolling sleeves up → Examiner may ask you to proceed with examination of just one elbow

Look	• Age & general physical condition of patient (BMI, frailty)
	• Disability aids
	• From front, sides & back
	  ○ Symmetry (compare sides)
	  ○ Carrying angle
	  ○ Deformity
	  ○ Stigmata of systemic disease
	  ○ Muscle wasting
	  ○ Scars
	  ○ Redness / swelling
		
		→ Normally 5–15°; increased = cubitus valgus; reduced = cubitus varus
		
		→ Psoriatic plaques, rheumatoid nodules
		
		→ Particularly olecranon bursitis

Feel	• Temperature – use back of hand & compare sides
	  ○ Medial elbow, posterior joint, lateral elbow
	• *"Tell me if I cause you any discomfort"*
	  ○ Palpate medial epicondyle
	  ○ Palpate around ulnar nerve behind medial epicondyle
	  ○ Palpate olecranon process
	  ○ Palpate lateral epicondyle
	  ○ Palpate radial head & radio-capitellar joint
	  ○ Palpate biceps tendon in antecubital fossa
		→ Warmth indicates inflammation
		
		→ Tender in medial (flexor) epicondylitis = 'Golfer's elbow'
		
		→ Tender in lateral (extensor) epicondylitis = 'Tennis elbow'
		→ If difficult to palpate, ask patient to pronate / supinate and feel for radial head pivoting under your fingers

Move	• Assess ROM and pain on movement
	• Active movement
	  ○ Looking from the side
	    ■ Flexion
	    ■ Extension
	  ○ Looking from in front with elbows flexed to 90° & tucked into sides
	    ■ Pronation
	    ■ Supination
	• Passive movement – *"Tell me if I cause you any discomfort"*
	  ○ Flexion / extension with your hand behind elbow
	  ○ Pronation / supination feeling radio-capitellar joint
		
		→ Normal 145°
		→ Normal 0° (females often able to hyperextend)
		
		→ Normally to at least 20° off fully palm-up
		→ Normally to at least 20° off fully palm-down
		→ Watch pt's face for evidence of discomfort
		→ Feel for crepitus

ELBOW

Special tests	• Resisted wrist flexion [⇨ Fig. 15]	→ Medial (flexor) epicondylitis = 'Golfer's elbow'
	o Ask patient to extend elbow & supinate forearm	
	o With one hand support elbow & palpate medial epicondyle	
	o With other hand passively extend the wrist	
	o Ask patient to try to flex wrist against resistance	
	o Pain over medial epicondyle = positive test	
	• Resisted wrist extension (Cozen's test) [⇨ Fig. 16]	→ Lateral (extensor) epicondylitis = 'Tennis elbow'
	o Ask patient to extend elbow, pronate forearm & make a fist	
	o With one hand support elbow & palpate lateral epicondyle	
	o "Cock your wrist back and keep it there"	
	o With your other hand push against the back of pt's hand, making them extend against resistance	
	o Pain over lateral epicondyle = positive test	
Function	• Both hands behind head	→ Washing hair, dressing
	• Both hands up to mouth	→ Eating
	• Both hands down to bottom	→ Cleaning after toilet
Neurovascular integrity	• Sensation	→ [p 54]
	o Median: lateral aspect of index finger	
	o Ulnar: medial aspect of little finger	
	o Radial: dorsal 1st interosseous space	
	• Radial pulse & CRT in finger	
Conclusion	• Wash / gel hands & thank pt	
	• If not done: "I would like to examine the other elbow"	
	• "I would like to examine the shoulder & wrist, then go on to complete a full musculoskeletal assessment"	
	• Investigations: X-rays (AP & lateral), MRI, joint aspiration	→ Joint above and below
		→ Pattern of joint involvement can aid diagnosis

ELBOW

Tennis & golfer's elbow

- Tennis elbow = extensor epicondylitis (lateral epicondyle)
- Golfer's elbow = flexor epicondylitis (medial epicondyle)
- Gradual onset of lateral (tennis) / medial (golfer's) elbow pain, often radiating into forearm
- Peak incidence age 40–50
- Tennis elbow is 5 times more common than Golfer's elbow
- Both are caused by repetitive, often strenuous activity
  - Sports (e.g. tennis / golf... either sport can cause either condition)
  - Heavy lifting
  - DIY
  - Gardening
  - Computer use
- Conservative management
  - Avoid activities that exacerbate symptoms
  - Analgesia & topical NSAIDs
  - Corticosteroid injections
  - Physiotherapy
  - Use of a forearm band orthosis
- Surgical tendon release is rarely required

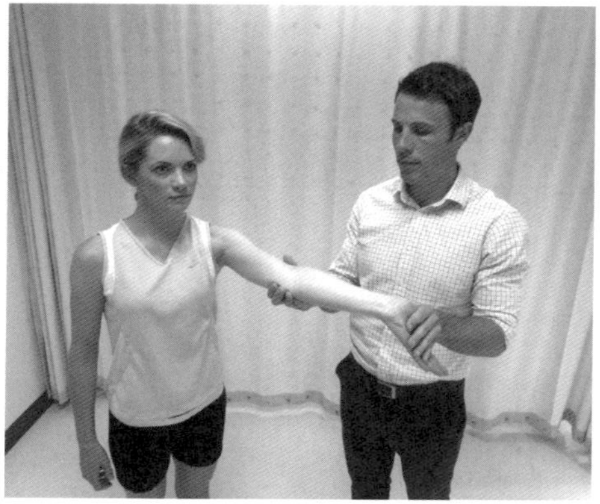

Fig. 15. Resisted wrist flexion. Medial (flexor) epicondylitis = 'Golfer's elbow'.

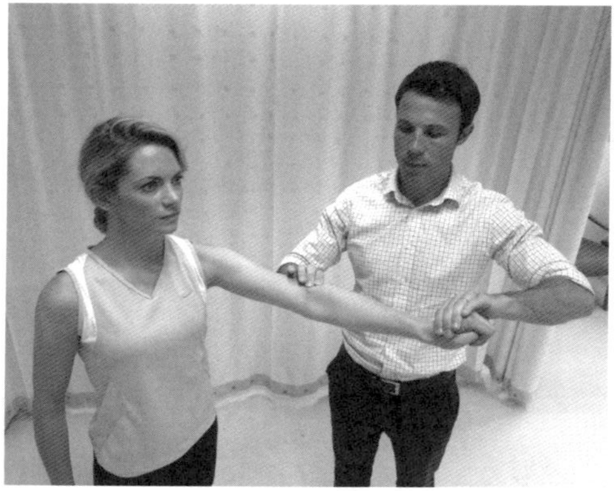

Fig. 16. Resisted wrist extension. Lateral (extensor) epicondylitis = 'Tennis elbow'.

ELBOW NOTES

NOTES

	Action / Examine for	ΔΔ / Potential findings / Extra information
Introduction	• Wash / gel hands • Introduce yourself, confirm pt, explain examination & gain consent • Expose & position pt (top off, standing) • "Do you have any pain in your back? Do you have any trouble walking?"	→ Consider chaperone

Look	• Age & general physical condition of pt (BMI, frailty)
	• Mobility aids
	• From front, sides and back
	  ○ Abnormal posture
	  ○ Muscle wasting
	  ○ Kyphosis
	  ○ Lordosis
	  ○ Scoliosis
		→ Crutches, walking sticks, wheelchair, etc
		
		→ Chronic back pain, RA
		→ Ankylosing spondylitis, osteoporotic #, RA
		→ Loss of lumbar lordosis in ankylosing spondylitis
		→ Idiopathic, neurofibromatosis

Feel	• Spinous processes (entire length of spine, cervical to lumbar) • Sacroiliac joints • Paraspinal muscles	→ Bony tenderness / abnormality → Sacroiliitis (e.g. ankylosing spondylitis) → Tenderness, spasm

Move	• Active movements only
	• Cervical spine
	  ○ Lateral flexion – "Try to touch your ear to your shoulder"
	  ○ Flexion – "Put your chin down onto your chest"
	  ○ Extension – "Put your head back as far as possible"
	  ○ Rotation – "Look over your shoulder"
	• Lumbar spine
	  ○ Flexion – "Try to touch your toes"
	  ○ Extension – "Lean back as far as possible"
	  ○ Lateral flexion – "Lean to side, slide your hand down your leg"
	• Thoracic spine
	  ○ Pt sitting on side of bed (stabilises pelvis)
	  ○ Rotation – "Twist your shoulders round"
		→ Passive movements are sometimes performed by specialists on the cervical spine, but are not included here

SPINE

Special tests

- Schober's test [➪ *Fig. 17*]
  - Pt standing, locate line between iliac crests (usually L3/4) → Around the same level as the dimples of Venus
  - Measure & mark spine 10 cm above and 5 cm below line with pen → Quantify lumbar spine flexion
  - Ask pt to bend forward with legs straight
  - Measure distance between marks at full flexion
  - >5 cm increase in distance is normal
  - <5 cm is abnormal
- Straight leg raise [➪ *Fig. 18*] → E.g. ankylosing spondylitis
  - Pt supine lying flat → L5 / S1 nerve root compression
  - *"Let me know if I cause you any pain"*
  - Holding ankle, keep leg straight and flex hip
  - Normally 90° of pain-free passive hip flexion should be possible
  - Back pain radiating down posterior leg = positive test
- Femoral stretch test [➪ *Fig. 19*] → L4 nerve root compression (note L1–L3 compression is rare)
  - Pt lying on front
  - *"Let me know if I cause you any pain"*
  - Hold thigh and ankle, keep leg straight and extend hip
  - Back pain radiating down anterior leg = positive test

Conclusion

- Wash / gel hands, thank pt, & allow to re-dress
- *"I would like to examine the rest of the musculoskeletal system"* → Pattern of joint involvement can aid diagnosis
- *"I would like to conduct a full neurological assessment of the lower limbs,* → Cauda equina syndrome, spinal cord compression
  and perform a digital rectal examination exam if indicated"
- Investigations: X-rays, MRI spine

SPINE

Ankylosing spondylitis

- Aetiology
  - Primary
  - Associated with psoriasis / IBD
- 5 males : 1 female (♂ usually severe disease)
- Presents in 20s
- Strong association with HLA-B27
- X-ray findings
  - Sacroiliitis
  - Bamboo spine
    - Squaring of vertebrae
    - Disc ossification
    - Spinal fusion (syndesmophytes)
  - Associated features
    - Uveitis
    - Peripheral enthesitis in 33% (especially Achilles tendonitis)
- Management
  - Simple analgesia
  - NSAIDs
  - Anti-TNFα therapy where NSAIDs fail

Neurogenic claudication

- Due to spinal stenosis (lumbosacral OA with narrowing of bony foramina & nerve root impingement)
- Calf / buttock / thigh discomfort when walking
- Classically relieved by bending forwards at waist (spinal flexion opens up bony foramina)
- This feature is useful in differentiating from intermittent (vascular) claudication

ΔΔ Lumbar back pain

- Mechanical
  - Muscular
  - Disc prolapse
  - OA
  - # (e.g. osteoporotic wedge #)
  - Spondylolisthesis (vertebral 'slipping')
  - Spinal stenosis
- Inflammatory
  - Ankylosing spondylitis
- Other serious pathology
  - Bone metastases
  - Myeloma
  - TB
  - Osteomyelitis

NOTES

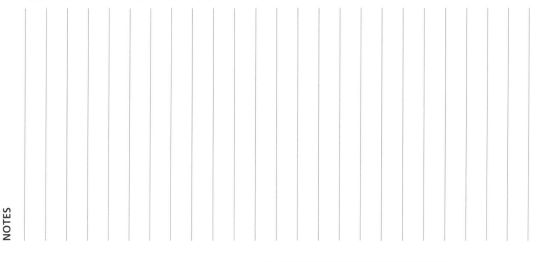

Fig. 17. **Schober's test.** Horizontal lines are drawn over top of iliac crests. Distance between marks should increase by at least 5 cm with normal lumbar spine flexion.

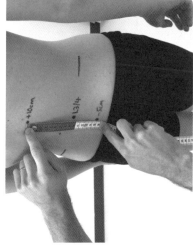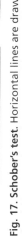

Fig. 18. **Straight leg raise.** L5/S1 nerve root compression. Watch the patient's face to identify pain.

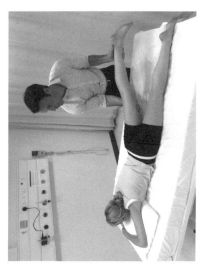

Fig. 19. **Femoral stretch test.** L4 nerve root compression.

Hand examination is common in OSCEs. There may be musculoskeletal pathology (e.g. rheumatoid, Dupuytren's), neurological pathology (e.g. ulnar nerve palsy), or signs related to other systemic disease (e.g. finger clubbing). Listen carefully to what you are asked to examine. If simply "examine this patient's hands" then follow this sequence, finishing with the neurological assessment described in the next section.

Action / Examine for	ΔΔ / Potential findings / Extra information
Introduction	
• Wash / gel hands	
• Introduce yourself, confirm pt, explain examination & gain consent	
• Expose & position pt (seated, exposed to above elbows, hands on a pillow)	
• *"Do you have any pain in your hands or arms?"*	
Look	
• Age & general physical condition of patient (BMI, frailty)	
• Disability aids	
• Palms facing down, start at nails & work proximally	
○ Nails	
■ Pitting, onycholysis	→ Psoriasis
■ Nailfold infarcts	→ Vasculitis, SLE
■ Finger clubbing, leuconychia, koilonychia	→ Other system pathology [p138]
○ Fingers	
■ Scars	→ Previous surgery for trauma / OA / RA
■ Swelling / erythema	→ Synovitis, infection
■ Swan-neck, boutonierre, Z-thumb	→ RA
■ Spindling	→ RA, scleroderma
■ Heberden's (DIP) & Bouchard's (PIP) nodes	→ OA – remember 'Outer *Heberdes*' = DIP
○ MCP joints	
■ Swelling / erythema	→ Synovitis, infection
■ Ulnar deviation	→ RA
■ Subluxation / dislocation	→ RA
○ Dorsum	
■ Tight, cold, waxy skin with telangectasia	→ Scleroderma
■ Interossei wasting	→ RA, ulnar nerve palsy
■ Rheumatoid nodules	→ RA
■ Psoriatic plaques	
○ Wrists	
■ Swelling / erythema	→ Synovitis, infection
■ Radiocarpal subluxation	→ RA
■ Prominent ulnar styloid	→ RA
• Turn hands over, palms facing up	
○ Flexion deformity of fingers	→ Dupuytren's, claw hand (ulnar nerve palsy, Klumpke's palsy)
○ Palms	
■ Scars	→ Dupuytren's release surgery
■ Thickening of palmar fascia	→ Dupuytren's
■ Wasting of thenar / hypothenar eminence	→ Median / ulnar nerve palsy
■ Palmar erythema	→ RA, CLD, hyperthyroidism, pregnancy
○ Wrists	
■ Scars	→ Carpal tunnel surgery
• Praying position (palms together, elbows up so wrists fully extended)	
○ Flexion deformity of fingers	→ RA, OA, scleroderma, Dupuytren's
• Make fists	
○ Loss of valleys between metacarpal heads due to MCPJ swelling	→ Synovitis

HANDS – GENERAL / MUSCULOSKELETAL

	• Hands up to chin to expose forearms / elbows
	  ○ Scars
	  ○ Rheumatoid nodules
	  ○ Psoriatic plaques
	• Ears, neck & scalp
	  ○ Psoriatic plaques
	  ○ Gouty tophi on ears
		→ Elbow trauma / surgery which may involve ulnar nerve
		→ RA
		
		→ Chronic tophaceous gout

Feel	• Temperature – use back of your hand & compare sides
	  ○ Dorsal MCP joints
	  ○ Dorsal wrists
	• Squeeze across joints, feeling for swelling / tenderness
	  ○ Wrists
	  ○ MCP joints
	  ○ Thumb interphalangeal joints
	  ○ General squeeze of other 4 fingers - if painful or abnormality identified on inspection assess individual finger joints in detail
	• Palpate for palmar fascia thickening
	• Assess any nodes / nodules
		→ Warmth indicates inflammation
		
		→ Synovitis, infection
		
		→ Dupuytren's
		→ [p94]

Move	• Assess ROM & pain on movement
	• Active movement
	  ○ Finger flexion (make fists) / extension
	  ○ Finger ABduction / ADduction
	  ○ Wrist flexion / extension / radial deviation / ulnar deviation
	  ○ Pronation / supination
	• Passive movement – *"Tell me if I cause you any discomfort"*
	  ○ Assess any joint that is abnormal (red, hot, swollen, deformed, reduced ROM on active movement)
		→ Watch pt's face for evidence of discomfort
		→ Inflamed joints (synovitis, infection) usually painful on passive movement

Function	• Pinch grip: *"Touch your thumb to each finger in turn"* • Power grip: *"Squeeze my fingers tightly"* • Fine motor control: do up a button, pick up a coin, pretend to play piano	

Neurovascular integrity	• Power / sensation / special tests
	  ○ Median
	  ○ Ulnar
	  ○ Radial
	• Radial pulse & CRT in fingers
		→ [p54]

Conclusion	• Wash/gel hands & thank pt • *"I would like to examine the elbows and shoulders, assess overall upper limb function then complete a full musculoskeletal assessment"* • Examine other relevant systems where relevant signs present • Investigations: X-ray, ESR / CRP, rheumatoid serology, joint aspiration	→ Pattern of joint involvement can aid diagnosis → e.g. finger clubbing, palmar erythema

HANDS – GENERAL / MUSCOLOSKELETAL

How to present your findings

In the common case of a pt with barn-door features of RA

- *"There is a symmetrical, deforming polyarthropathy affecting the small joints of the hands in a rheumatoid pattern. The most common differentials for this clinical picture are RA and psoriatic arthropathy."*

'**Examine this pt's hands' cases – modify your examination based on what you find**

- Musculoskeletal: OA, RA, psoriatic arthropathy, gout, Dupuytren's contracture
- Neurological: Median nerve palsy (carpal tunnel), radial nerve palsy, ulnar nerve palsy (check for elbow trauma), T1 lesion, MND
- Endocrine: Thyroid disease, acromegaly
- Other: Finger clubbing, scleroderma, leuconychia, koilonychia

RA statistics

- 3 females : 1 male
- Peak prevalence age 30–50
- 70% seropositive (as is 5% of general population)
  - Rheumatoid factor +ve (IgM against self-IgG)
  - Often have nodules
  - Extra-articular features
  - Progressive disease
- 20% of all RA pts have nodules
- 50% HLA-DR4 +ve (severe, erosive disease)

Extra-articular features of RA

- General: Malaise, lethargy, low grade fever, weight loss
- CVS: Pericarditis, pericardial effusion
- RS: Nodules, pleural effusion, pulmonary fibrosis, pneumoconiosis (Caplan's syndrome)
- GUS: Renal amyloid
- NS: Polyneuropathy, mononeuritis multiplex, carpal tunnel, atlanto-axial subluxation
- Eyes: Scleritis, episcleritis, keratoconjunctivitis sicca, Sjögren's syndrome
- Blood: Anaemia [see below], thrombocytosis, ↓WCC (Felty's syndrome = ↓WCC + splenomegaly + RA)

Features of *active* RA

- Inflamed joints
  - Red
  - Hot
  - Swollen
  - Tender
- Pain on passive movement
- Increased duration of morning stiffness
- Raised ESR
- Anaemia [see below]

Multifactorial aetiology of anaemia in RA
- Anaemia of chronic disease
- Iron deficiency anaemia secondary to NSAID-induced gastritis / peptic ulcer
- Aplastic anaemia secondary to DMARD
- Macrocytic anaemia secondary to methotrexate (folate metabolism)
- Pernicious anaemia (associated with RA)

RA X-ray
- Loss of joint space
- Bony erosions
- Periarticular osteoporosis
- Deformity (e.g. subluxation)
- Soft tissue swelling

OA X-ray
- Loss of joint space
- Osteophytes
- Subchondral sclerosis
- Bone cysts

Psoriatic arthropathy
- Affects 10% of pts with psoriasis
- In 75% skin features present before arthropathy
- In 20% skin features present after arthropathy
- In 5% no skin features will ever appear

Presentations of psoriatic arthropathy
- Asymmetrical oligoarthritis
  - Mainly hands and feet (dactylitis)
  - Sometimes larger joints
- Lone DIP disease
- Rheumatoid pattern
- Arthritis mutilans
- Sacroiliitis

Sjögren's syndrome
- May occur independently
- May be associated with RA / SLE / scleroderma
- Features
  - Dry eyes (keratoconjunctivitis sicca)
  - Dry mouth (xerostomia)
  - Parotid gland enlargement

DMARDs & key side effects
- All DMARDS
  - Marrow suppression
  - Hepatotoxicity
  - Rash
  - GI upset (especially nausea & oral ulcers)
- Methotrexate
  - Pneumonitis & pulmonary fibrosis [p13]
  - Megalobastic anaemia
- Hydroxychloroquine
  - Retinopathy
- Sulfasalazine
  - Oligospermia
- IM Gold
  - Nephrotic syndrome
- Penicillamine
  - Nephrotic syndrome
  - Altered taste
  - Myasthenia gravis-like syndrome
- Ciclosporin
  - Renal impairment
  - HTN
  - Gum hypertrophy
- Leflunomide
- Azathioprine

NOTES

Neurological assessment of the hands may be performed in isolation or following musculoskeletal examination [p50]. You may be asked to examine a single nerve, or all 3 at once: *"Examine the nerves supplying the hand"*. If all 3, it is probably slicker to do all the inspection first, then power testing and so on, working through the 3 nerves each time. Practice all possible scenarios so you can cope with whatever the examiner throws at you.

	Action / Examine for	ΔΔ / Potential findings / Extra information
Introduction	• Wash / gel hands • Introduce yourself, confirm pt, explain examination & gain consent • Expose (hands & arms up to elbows at least) • *"Do you have any pain, tingling or weakness in your arms or hands?"*	

Median nerve		

Inspection	• Wasting of thenar eminence
	  ○ Pt in 'begging' position, hands together with palms up
	  ○ Compare sides
	• Carpal tunnel decompression scar (palm / wrist)
		→ Much easier to identify wasting when comparing sides

Power	• Thumb ABduction
	  ○ Palm facing upwards
	  ○ *"Point your thumb straight up towards your nose"*
	  ○ With one finger, push thumb back towards palm
	  ○ *"Don't let me push your thumb down"*
		→ Tests ABductor pollicis brevis [LOAF ⇔]
		There are other ways of testing median nerve motor function (e.g. opponens pollicis), but this is a common method and easy to perform

Sensation	• Test lateral side of index finger
	  ○ Ask pt to close eyes
	  ○ *"Say yes when you feel me touch your skin"*
	  ○ *"Does that feel normal? Is it the same on both sides?"*
		→ [⇔ *Fig. 20*]

Special tests	• Tinel test
	  ○ Repeatedly percuss over the carpal tunnel (ventral wrist)
	  ○ Paraesthesia in the median distribution = positive test
	• Phalen test
	  ○ Wrist held in flexion for 30–60 sec
	  ○ Paraesthesia in median distribution = positive test
		→ Carpal tunnel syndrome
		
		→ Carpal tunnel syndrome

HANDS – NEUROLOGICAL

Ulnar nerve		

Inspection	• Wasting of hypothenar eminence
	  ○ Pt in 'begging' position, hands together
	  ○ Compare sides
	• Backs of hands for wasting of interossei (especially 1st)
	• Partial claw hand
	  ○ Weak medial lumbricals – clawing of little and ring fingers
	  ○ Lateral lumbricals unaffected (median innervation)
	• Check elbows
	  ○ Scars
	  ○ Evidence of trauma / deformity
		→ Skin 'sinking' between tendons
		  [↳ Fig. 22]
		→ [LOAF ↻]

Power	• Finger ABduction
	  ○ Palm facing downwards
	  ○ Hold digits 3–5 between your thumb and fingers
	  ○ ABduct the pt's index finger for them
	  ○ With one finger push index finger back across towards 3rd finger
	  ○ "Don't let me push your finger in"
		→ [↳ Fig. 21]
		→ Testing ABduction purely in the index finger rather than across all fingers is more sensitive and looks slicker

Sensation	• Test medial side of little finger (method as above)	→ [↳ Fig. 20]

Special tests	• Froment's sign
	  ○ Ask pt to pinch paper between a straight thumb and index finger
	  ○ Instruct to grip paper as you pull it away
	  ○ Flexed DIP joint of thumb = positive test
		→ [↳ Fig. 23]
		→ Long thumb flexors used to compensate for weak ADductor pollicis

Radial nerve		
Inspection	• Wrist drop • (Note: No wasting in hand – no intrinsic muscles supplied by radial nerve)	→ ΔΔ C7 radiculopathy [↻]
Power	• Wrist extension • Finger extension	
Sensation	• Test dorsal 1st interosseous space (method as above)	→ [↳ Fig. 20]
Special tests	–	

| Conclusion | • Wash / gel hands and thank pt
• "I would like to examine the rest of the upper limb neurology, then go on to complete a full neurological examination"
• Investigations: Nerve conduction studies | |

HANDS – NEUROLOGICAL

Features of palsy		Median nerve	Ulnar nerve	Radial nerve
Sensory innervation		Lateral palm Thumb & lateral 2½ fingers	Medial hand (palm & dorsum) Medial 1½ fingers	Lateral dorsum of hand (no fingers)
Motor innervation		**LOAF** muscles of hand • Lateral 2 lumbricals • Opponens pollicis • ABductor pollicis brevis • Flexor pollicis brevis	Small muscles of the hand with the exception of the LOAF muscles	Extensors • Fingers • Wrist • Elbow
Mechanism of injury		Carpal tunnel syndrome	Elbow (funny bone) trauma Hand trauma (*rare*)	Humeral shaft # Saturday night palsy*
	Wasting	Thenar eminence	Hypothenar eminence Interossei (1st most obvious)	–
	Posture	–	Partial claw hand	Wrist drop
	Sensory	Pain / sensory loss as above	Pain / sensory loss as above	Pain / sensory loss as above
	Motor	Weak thumb ABduction	Weak finger ABduction	Weak finger / wrist extension
	Tests	Tinel / Phalen +ve	Froment's sign	–

Note that a C7 radiculopathy causes a similar motor deficit to radial nerve palsy, but with sensory loss in the index and middle fingers rather than on the dorsal 1st interosseous space [see diagram on p60]

T_1 lesion
- Aetiology
  - Cervical spondylosis
  - Pancoast tumour
  - Plexus trauma / birth injury (Klumpke's palsy)
- Clinical features
  - Total claw hand (all lumbricals lost)
  - Wasting of small muscles in hand
  - Pain / sensory loss in medial forearm
  - Horner's syndrome may co-exist

ΔΔ **Carpal tunnel syndrome**
- Idiopathic (majority of case)
- Pregnancy
- RA
- Hypothyroid
- Diabetes
- Acromegaly

* Saturday night palsy = compression of the radial nerve against the humerus by falling asleep with your arm over the back of a chair

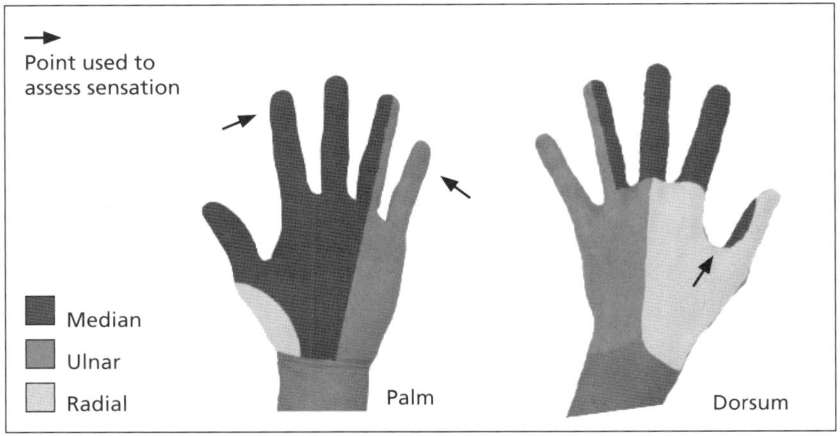

Patient is asked to hold piece of paper between index finger and a *straight* thumb

Paper is then pulled away from patient:

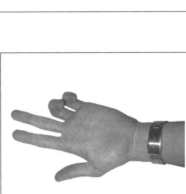
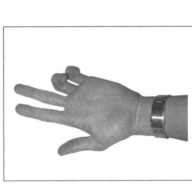

Normal function
(Thumb DIP joint remains extended)

Froment's sign
(Thumb DIP joint flexes as long flexors compensate for ADductor pollicis weakness)

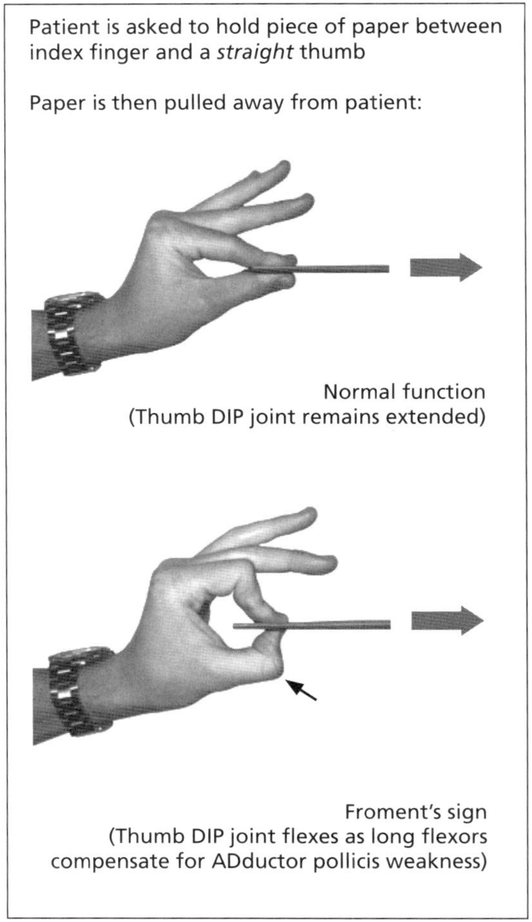

Fig. 23. Froment's sign (Ulnar palsy)

Point used to assess sensation

Dorsum

Palm

Median
Ulnar
Radial

Fig. 20. Sensory innervation of the left hand by the peripheral nerves

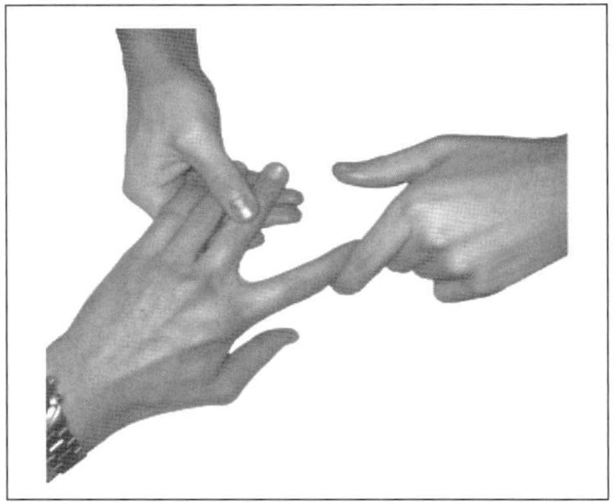

Fig. 22. Partial claw hand (Ulnar palsy)

Fig. 21. Assessment of finger ABduction (Ulnar nerve)

	Action / Examine for	ΔΔ / Potential findings / Extra information
Introduction	• Wash / gel hands • Introduce yourself, confirm pt, explain examination & gain consent • Expose & position pt (top off, supine at 45°) • *"Do you have any pain, tingling or weakness in your arms or hands?"*	→ Consider chaperone

Inspection	• Symmetry, muscle wasting, fasciculation
	• Abnormal posturing
	  ○ UMN posture (shoulder ADducted, elbow/wrist flexed, pronated)
	  ○ Erb's palsy (waiter's tip)
	• Pronator drift
	  ○ Ask pt to stretch arms out in front of them, palms facing upwards
	  ○ *"Close your eyes, and keep your arms there"*
	  ○ If hand drifts down and pronates – positive result on that side
		→ Wasting & fasciculation = LMN
		
		→ UMN lesion (e.g. stroke)
		→ [↔]
		→ Subtle UMN weakness (e.g. stroke)
		→ If pt cannot do this then you don't need to do the test (i.e. weakness is already obvious)

Tone	• Take pt's hand in 'shaking hands' grip, supporting arm at elbow • *"Let your arm go totally floppy"* • Pronate / supinate to detect supinator catch • Flex / extend wrist • Flex / extend elbow • *"Tap your knee with your other hand"* – continue to flex / extend elbow • Repeat with the other arm	→ Early sign of increased tone → 'Clasp-knife' hypertonia = UMN lesion → Synkinesis (reinforces hypertonia)
Power	• *"Are you right- or left-handed?"* • Ask pt to 'push me away' or 'pull me towards you' where possible • Assess each movement on one side then compare with the other • Grade power out of 5 | Movement	Root	Nerve | |---|---|---| | Shoulder ABduction* | C5 | Axillary | | Elbow flexion | C5 / C6 | Musculocutaneous | | Elbow extension* | C7 | Radial | | Wrist extension* | C6 | Radial | | Finger extension* | C7 | Radial | | Finger flexion | C8 | Median + ulnar | | Thumb ABduction | T1 | Median | | Finger ABduction | T1 | Ulnar |	→ Can influence power in arms → Isotonic testing = more sensitive → [↔] → Not all movements need testing – these cover all roots, nerves & joints The main thing is to identify any deficit present. Working out whether the pattern if involvement is related to a root or peripheral nerve issue can be difficult and time consuming, and history/context is often key *Weak in UMN lesion
Reflexes	• Ask pt to relax and close their eyes | Reflex	Root | |---|---| | Biceps jerk | C5 / C6 | | Triceps jerk | C7 | | Supinator jerk | C5 / C6 |	→ If difficulty relaxing, ask to clench teeth immediately before striking tendon → Strike thumb placed on tendon → Strike directly → Strike directly

UPPER LIMB NEUROLOGY

Co-ordination	• 'Piano playing' – hold hands out and wiggle fingers	→ Difficult in UMN lesion, Parkinson's
	• Hand slapping test for dysdiadokinesis [p78]	→ Cerebellar ataxia
	• Finger–nose test [p78]	→ Cerebellar ataxia
Sensation	• Light touch (cotton wool) then pain (neurotip)	
	○ Ask pt to close eyes, demonstrate on their sternum (midline)	→ Never assess with eyes open – pt may see you touch skin and say they feel it regardless
	○ "Say yes when you feel me touch your skin"	
	○ Move from side to side – "Does it feel the same on both sides?"	
		→ [↔ for diagram]

Area	Root
Above shoulder tip	C4
Regimental badge area	C5
Tip of thumb	C6
Tip of middle finger	C7
Tip of little finger	C8
Medial mid-forearm	T1

	• Assess peripheral nerve dermatomes if nerve rather than root problem suspected	→ Radial/median/ulnar in hand [p54] & others more proximal
	• Sensory level on arms if peripheral neuropathy suspected	→ 'Glove and stocking' sensory loss (e.g. diabetic neuropathy)
	○ Tap cotton wool up arm starting at tip of middle finger	
	○ Ask pt to tell you when they feel sensation *change*	
	○ Repeat on other arm	
	• Joint position sense	
	○ Use middle finger DIP joint	
	○ Immobilise middle phalanx with one hand, hold distal finger by sides	→ Avoid touching finger pulp as this allows touch to be used, rather than simply joint position sense
	○ "Close your eyes and tell me if your finger is up, down or if you're not sure"	
	○ Randomly move finger tip up/down & ask pt its position 3–4 times	
	○ Repeat on other arm	
	• Vibration sense	→ Lost early in peripheral neuropathy
	○ Ask pt to close eyes	
	○ "Tell me if you feel buzzing or pushing"	
	○ Strike tuning fork to make it vibrate	→ Crude touch may be retained though vibration sense is lost
	○ Hold heel of tuning fork to middle finger tip → radial styloid → olecranon → shoulder tip	→ No need to move proximally if vibration is perceived distally
	○ Repeat on other arm	
	• (Temperature – rarely formally assessed)	
Conclusion	• Wash / gel hands, thank pt & allow them to re-dress	
	• "I would like to perform a more detailed examination of the neurology of the hands, then go on to complete a full neurological examination"	→ [p54]
	• Investigations: Nerve conduction studies, imaging (CT / MRI)	

UPPER LIMB NEUROLOGY

Clinical features of LMN lesion, UMN lesion, extrapyramidal pathology & cerebellar lesion

	LMN lesion	UMN lesion	Extrapyramidal [p74]	Cerebellar lesion [p78]
Tone	Normal or ↓	↑ (spastic)	↑ (rigid)	→
Power	↓	→	Normal	Normal
Reflexes	Reduced	Brisk	Normal	Normal
Plantars	Down	Up	Down	Down
Co-ordination	Normal	→	→	→
Other features	Wasting Fasciculation	Clonus	Resting tremor Bradykinesia Postural instability	Intention tremor Nystagmus Cerebellar speech

MRC Scale.

Grading of power (0–5)

5 Normal
   Full power against resistance

4 Reduced power
   Able to move against some resistance

3 Able to move against gravity
   Unable to move against resistance

2 Unable to move against gravity
   Able to move if gravity eliminated (e.g. can ABduct shoulder when lying supine but not when standing)

1 Visible flicker of muscle contraction but no movement across joint

0 No muscle contraction

Suggested points for assessing sensation (nerve root dermatomes C4–T1)

Right arm anterior view

C4: above shoulder tip

C5: regimental badge area

C6: tip of thumb

C7: tip of middle finger

C8: tip of little finger

T1: medial mid-forearm

UPPER LIMB NEUROLOGY NOTES

Sensory modalities carried in the spinal cord

- Spinothalamic tracts
  - Pain
  - Temperature
  - Crude touch
- Dorsal columns
  - Vibration
  - Joint position sense
  - Fine touch

Pathology of spinal cord sensory tracts

- Spinothalamic
  - Syringomyelia
  - Anterior spinal artery occlusion
- Dorsal columns
  - Tabes dorsalis (syphilis)
  - SCDC [p65]
- Any
  - MS

Syringomyelia

- Expansion of spinal cord central canal due to CSF blockage (commonly Chiari malformation)
- Spinothalamic fibres principally affected
- Loss of pain & temperature sensation in 'cape-like' distribution over arms, shoulders & upper body
- LMN signs in upper limbs, spastic paraparesis of lower limbs
- Dorsal column signs develop as canal (syrinx) further expands
- Syringobulbia if syrinx extends into brainstem [p73]

Brachial plexus injuries at birth

	Erb's palsy	Klumpke's palsy
Part of plexus injured	Upper plexus (C5–C7)	Lower plexus (C8–T1)
Mechanism of injury	Shoulder dystocia during birth	Excessive arm traction during birth
Clinical features	Sensory loss down lateral arm 'Waiter's tip' position • Shoulder ADducted • Elbow extended • Arm internally rotated • Forearm pronated	Sensory loss in medial forearm & hand Complete claw hand Wasting of small muscles in hand Horner's syndrome may co-exist

NOTES

	Action / Examine for	ΔΔ / Potential findings / Extra information
Introduction	• Wash / gel hands • Introduce yourself, confirm pt, explain examination & gain consent • Expose & position pt (pants / shorts only, supine) • *"Do you have any pain, tingling or weakness in your legs or feet?"*	→ Consider chaperone *Examine feet!* *gait!*

Inspection	• Symmetry, muscle wasting, fasciculation
	• Abnormal posturing
	  ○ UMN posture (hip / knee extended, foot plantarflexed and inverted)
	  ○ Foot drop
	• Soft tissue damage due to sensory neuropathy (especially feet)
		→ Wasting & fasciculation = LMN
		→ UMN lesion (e.g. stroke)
		→ [↔]
		→ Blisters, ulcers, Charcot joints [p36]

Tone	• *"Let your leg go totally floppy"* • Rock leg from side to side • Suddenly pull upwards from behind knee – if leg stays straight (and heel comes off bed) this indicates hypertonia • Suddenly pull each foot into dorsiflexion to elicit clonus (3+ beats)	→ Don't be too rough with the pt! → UMN lesion
Power	• Ask pt to 'push me away' or 'pull me towards you' where possible • Assess each movement on one side then compare with the other • Grade power out of 5	→ 'Isotonic' testing = more sensitive → [p60]

Movement	Root	Nerve
Hip flexion	L1 / L2	Femoral
Hip extension (push heel into bed)	L5 / S1	Gluteal
Knee flexion	L5 / S1	Sciatic
Knee extension	L3 / L4	Femoral
Ankle dorsiflexion	L4	Peroneal
Big toe extension	L5	Peroneal
Ankle plantarflexion	S1	Tibial

The main thing is to identify any deficit present; working out whether the pattern of involvement is related to a root or peripheral nerve issue can be difficult and time consuming, and history / context is often key

→ Hence foot drop with common peroneal nerve injury (e.g. proximal fibula #)

Reflexes	• Ask pt to relax and close their eyes	→ If difficulty relaxing, ask to clench teeth immediately before you strike the tendon

Reflex	Root
Knee jerk (palpate tendon first)	L3 / L4
Ankle jerk	S1

• Plantar reflexes
  ○ Run thumb nail up lateral side of foot, watch hallux
  ○ Up / down / equivocal

→ Different methods – choose one you like & become slick at it
→ *First movement of hallux counts*
→ Up (+ve Babinski) = UMN lesion

Co-ordination	• Heel–shin test [p79]	→ Cerebellar ataxia

Sensation	• Light touch (cotton wool) then pain (neurotip)
	  ○ Ask pt to close eyes, demonstrate on their sternum (midline)
	  ○ *"Say yes when you feel me touch your skin"*
	  ○ Move from side to side – *"Does it feel the same on both sides?"*
		→ Never assess with eyes open – pt may see you touch skin and say they feel it regardless

LOWER LIMB NEUROLOGY

Sensation

Area	Root	[↪ for diagram]
Antero-medial mid thigh	L2	
Medial thigh just above knee	L3	
Medial malleolus	L4	
Dorsal 1st web space	L5	
Lateral heel	S1	

- Assess peripheral nerve dermatomes if nerve rather than root problem suspected
- Sensory level on legs if peripheral neuropathy suspected → 'Glove and stocking' sensory loss (e.g. diabetic neuropathy)
  - Tap cotton wool up antero-medial leg starting at tip of hallux
  - Ask pt to tell you when they feel sensation *change*
  - Repeat on other leg
- Joint position sense (proprioception)
  - Use hallux
  - Immobilize forefoot with one hand; hold distal hallux at sides → Avoid touching pulp of hallux as this allows touch to be used, rather than simply joint position sense
  - *"Close your eyes and tell me when your big toe is up, down, or if you're not sure"*
  - Randomly move hallux up/down & ask pt its position 3–4 times
  - Repeat on other foot
- Vibration sense
  - *"Close your eyes and tell me if you feel buzzing or pushing"*
  - Strike tuning fork to make it vibrate → Lost early in peripheral neuropathy / Crude touch may be retained though vibration sense is lost
  - Hold base of fork to pulp of hallux → medial malleolus → tibial tuberosity → ASIS → No need to move proximally if vibration is perceived distally
  - Repeat on other leg
  - (Temperature – rarely formally assessed)

Special tests

- Romberg's test → Sensory ataxia due to proprioceptive loss [↔] / May be impossible if legs very weak
  - Stand pt up, feet together, facing you
  - Hover your hands above pt's shoulders
  - *"Now close your eyes. I will catch you if necessary"* → Without visual input and with impaired proprioception pt cannot maintain balance
  - If pt suddenly becomes very unsteady – positive test
  - Steady pt's shoulders and instruct to open eyes
- Straight leg raise [p47] → L5 / S1 nerve root impingement
- Femoral stretch test [p47] → L4 nerve root impingement

Conclusion

- Wash / gel hands, thank pt & allow them to re-dress
- *"I would now like to assess gait then complete a full neurological examination"* → [p22]
- Spastic paraparesis: examine for sensory level on thorax
- Flaccid paraparesis: perform PR & check for saddle anaesthesia → Cauda equina syndrome
- Investigations: nerve conduction studies / CT head / MRI spine

Romberg reg at least 2 of:
1) Proprioception - DCML
2) Vestibular function
3) Vision.

LOWER LIMB NEUROLOGY

Suggested points for assessing sensation (nerve root dermatomes L2–S1)

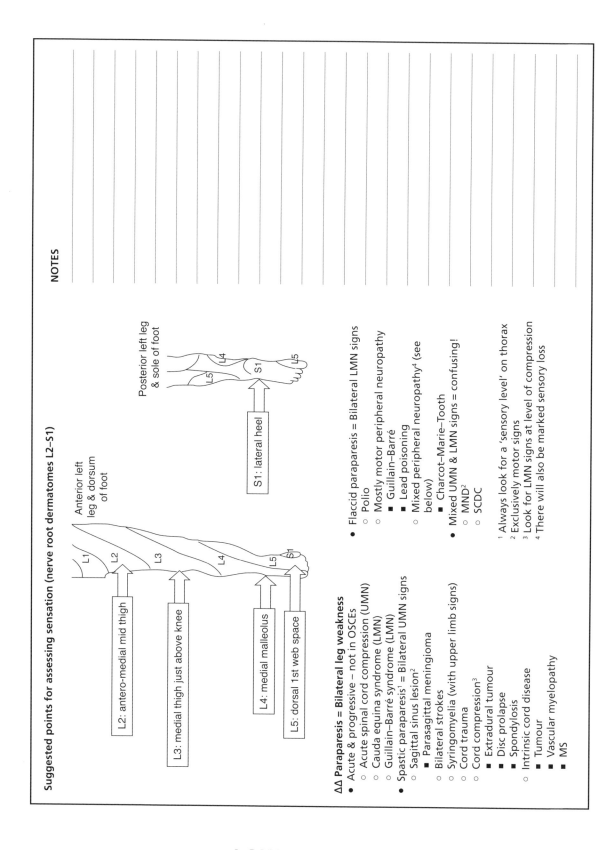

Anterior left leg & dorsum of foot

Posterior left leg & sole of foot

L2: antero-medial mid thigh

L3: medial thigh just above knee

L4: medial malleolus

L5: dorsal 1st web space

S1: lateral heel

ΔΔ Paraparesis = Bilateral leg weakness

- Acute & progressive – not in OSCEs
  - ○ Acute spinal cord compression (UMN)
  - ○ Cauda equina syndrome (LMN)
  - ○ Guillain–Barré syndrome (LMN)
- Spastic paraparesis[1] = Bilateral UMN signs
  - ○ Sagittal sinus lesion[2]
    - ▪ Parasagittal meningioma
  - ○ Bilateral strokes
  - ○ Syringomyelia (with upper limb signs)
  - ○ Cord trauma
  - ○ Cord compression[3]
    - ▪ Extradural tumour
    - ▪ Disc prolapse
    - ▪ Spondylosis
  - ○ Intrinsic cord disease
    - ▪ Tumour
    - ▪ Vascular myelopathy
    - ▪ MS

- Flaccid paraparesis = Bilateral LMN signs
  - ○ Polio
  - ○ Mostly motor peripheral neuropathy
    - ▪ Guillain–Barré
    - ▪ Lead poisoning
  - ○ Mixed peripheral neuropathy[4] (see below)
    - ▪ Charcot–Marie–Tooth
- Mixed UMN & LMN signs = confusing!
  - ○ MND[2]
  - ○ SCDC

[1] Always look for a 'sensory level' on thorax
[2] Exclusively motor signs
[3] Look for LMN signs at level of compression
[4] There will also be marked sensory loss

ΔΔ Unilateral leg weakness
- UMN
  - Stroke
  - Tumour
  - MS
- LMN
  - Root lesion
  - Nerve lesion

ΔΔ Peripheral neuropathy
- Mostly sensory
  - Diabetes mellitus
  - Uraemia (renal failure)
- Mostly motor
  - Guillain–Barré
  - Lead poisoning
- Mixed
  - Charcot–Marie–Tooth
  - B12 / folate deficiency (also cause SCDC)
  - Thiamine deficiency
  - Alcohol
  - Vasculitis / SLE
  - Paraneoplastic
  - Amyloid

Positive Romberg's test (sensory ataxia)
- Dorsal column loss
  - Tabes dorsalis (syphilis)
  - SCDC
  - MS
- Sensory peripheral neuropathy

[see relevant information p60]
- Clinical features of UMN lesion, LMN lesion, extrapyramidal pathology and cerebellar lesion
- System used for grading of power
- Sensory modalities in the spinal cord

SCDC (B$_{12}$ / folate deficiency)
- Spastic paraparesis
- Upgoing plantars
- Reduced knee jerks
- Loss of ankle jerks
- Dorsal column loss
  - Loss of vibration sense
  - Loss of joint position sense
  - Sensory ataxia (+ve Romberg's)

MND can cause almost any collection of motor signs

Amyotrophic lateral sclerosis (type of MND)
- Weakness
- Wasting   } LMN signs
- Fasciculation
- Spasticity   } UMN signs
- Brisk reflexes

ΔΔ Foot drop
- Common peroneal nerve palsy
- Stroke
- L4 / L5 root lesion
- MND
- Charcot–Marie–Tooth syndrome [p36]

NOTES

Introduction		• Wash / gel hands • Introduce yourself, confirm pt, explain examination & gain consent • Position pt (sitting opposite you, 1–2 m away with your heads at roughly the same level)

	Attribute	**Method of examination**	**ΔΔ / Potential findings / Extra information**
I Olfactory	Smell	• *"Have you noticed any changes in your sense of smell?"*	
II Optic	Visual acuity	• *"Do you wear glasses or contact lenses?"* • *"Have you had any problems with your vision recently?"* • Ask pt to read something, covering one eye at a time • Indicate you would ideally use a Snellen chart at 6 m	→ A common mistake is to allow pt to use both eyes at once

	Visual fields	• Inattention
		  ○ *"Look at my nose"*
		  ○ Put your arms directly out to sides, pointing fingers
		  ○ *"Keep looking at my nose; point to the finger I move"*
		  ○ Wiggle left, right, then both fingers at once
		• Visual fields (ideally use white hat pin)
		  ○ *"Look at my nose; can you see my whole face?"*
		  ○ Ask pt to cover left eye with left hand
		  ○ *"With your right eye, look into my left eye"*
		  ○ Close / cover your own right eye
		  ○ *"Keep looking into my eye and tell me when you see the white dot out of the corner of your eye"*
		  ○ Move hat pin towards centre from 4 corners of visual field
		  ○ Compare pt's visual fields with your own
		  ○ Repeat on pt's right eye
			→ Usually the result of a stroke
			
			→ Pt with inattention will only see one finger move
			
			→ Crude assessment of fields
			
			→ Closing rather than covering your eye frees both your arms to slickly manoeuvre the hat pin
			
			→ Top left, bottom left, top right, bottom right

	Pupillary reflexes
	(also CN III)
		• Ask pt to concentrate on a spot on the wall
		• *"I am going to briefly shine my torch into your eyes"*
		• Look for direct & consensual responses
		• Swinging torch test
		  ○ Repeatedly 'swing' torch between eyes
		  ○ Look for inappropriate pupillary dilation when light shone at that eye
			→ RAPD (Marcus Gunn pupil)
			→ Shine in left eye for 1 sec, right eye for 1 sec & keep repeating

	Fundus	• *"Ideally I would like to examine the fundus by ophthalmoscopy"*	

CRANIAL NERVES

III Oculomotor IV Trochlear VI Abducens	Eye movements	• Note any ptosis & abnormal position of eye	→ e.g. CN III palsy
		• "Keep your head still and follow my finger with your eyes"	→ This is essential
		• "Tell me if you see double at any point"	
		• Finger at least 50 cm from face, move slowly in an 'H' pattern	
		• Look for obvious ophthalmoplegia & nystagmus	
		• If suggestion of nystagmus, move finger more quickly to elicit	→ Slight nystagmus at extremes of lateral gaze occurs in some normal individuals
		• If there is diplopia	
		○ Ask if images separated horizontally or vertically	→ Should allow identification of ophthalmoplegic eye but can be difficult for pt
		○ Cover each eye in turn, which image disappears?	
		○ Looking to side – lateral image from affected eye	
		○ Looking down – lower image from affected eye	
		○ Looking up – upper image from affected eye	
	Accommodation	• "Keep looking at my finger"	
		• Move finger slowly in towards pt's nose	
		• Check that pupils constrict appropriately during convergence	→ Note that convergence is preserved in INO [p72]

V Trigeminal	Sensory	• Ask pt to close eyes	
		• "Say 'yes' when you feel me touching your face"	
		• Move from side to side: "Does it feel the same on both sides?"	→ You could assess pain (neurotip) and light touch (cotton wool) sensation here if time
		○ Ophthalmic division: above eyebrows	
		○ Maxillary division: over zygoma	
		○ Mandibular division: chin either side of the midline	
	Motor	• Jaw opening against resistance	→ Pterygoid muscles
		○ Push upwards on bottom of pt's chin	
		○ "Open your jaw against my hand"	
		○ Jaw will deviate towards side of weakness	
		• Jaw clenching	→ Masseter muscles
		○ Palpate for masseter contraction above angle of jaw	
	Reflexes	• Corneal reflex	→ Same branch of trigeminal is implicated in nostril sensation and corneal reflex
		○ Can be assessed indirectly	
		○ Test sensation inside nostrils with wisp of cotton wool	
		• Jaw jerk	
		○ "Let your mouth hang open"	
		○ Place your thumb on pt's chin	
		○ "I'm going to tap your chin, keep your mouth open and relaxed"	
		○ Strike thumb briskly with tendon hammer	
		■ Minimal / absent = normal	
		■ Brisk = UMN lesion	→ Stroke / tumour / MS, etc.

CRANIAL NERVES

	Attribute	Method of examination	ΔΔ / Potential findings / Extra info

VII Facial	Facial tone	• Look for signs of reduced facial tone
		   ○ Reduced wrinkling of forehead
		   ○ Drooping of corner of mouth
		   ○ Flattening of the nasolabial fold
			→ Occurs in LMN facial nerve lesions only [↬]

	Motor	• Raise eyebrows
		• Screw up eyes
		   ○ *"Keep them tightly shut"* – try to pull open
		   ○ Bell's sign = upgaze on attempted eye closure
		• Puff out cheeks
		• Show gums
			→ Facial nerve (e.g. Bell's) palsy

	Sensory	• Chorda tympani – supplies anterior $^2/_3$ of tongue
		   ○ *"Have you noticed any change in taste?"*
		• Branch to stapedius
		   ○ *"Are you troubled by loud noises?"*	

VIII Vestibulo-cochlear	Hearing	• Stroke tragus or occlude external auditory meatus of one ear • Ask pt to repeat numbers you whisper in their other ear • Change sides and repeat	→ Crude assessment of hearing

	Special tests	• Rinne test
		   ○ Assess each ear in turn
		   ○ First place heel of vibrating tuning fork on mastoid process behind ear
		     – *"This is sound number one"*
		   ○ Secondly place prongs of vibrating tuning fork close to (but not touching) the external auditory meatus – *"This is sound number two"*
		     "Which was louder, sound one or two?"
		• Weber test
		   ○ Place heel of vibrating tuning fork in centre of pt's forehead
		   ○ *"Do you hear the sound more on the left or right, or just in the middle of your head?"*
			→ [↬ for interpretation]
			
			→ Bone conduction
			
			→ Air conduction
			
			→ [↬ for interpretation]

CRANIAL NERVES

IX	Glosso-pharyngeal	Bulbar function	• Soft palate movement
			○ Shine pen torch in mouth
X	Vagus		○ "Say 'ahhh' please"
XII	Hypoglossal		○ Look at movement of uvula
			○ Pulled away from side of weakness
			• Speech
			• Swallowing water

→ Generally assessed throughout examination
→ Choking / spluttering = possible bulbar deficit

		Tongue	• Appearance
			○ Normal
			○ Flaccid, wasted & fasciculating
			○ Spastic & contracted
			• Movements
			○ "Stick your tongue straight out"
			○ Deviates towards side of weakness
			○ "Move your tongue from side to side"

→ Bulbar palsy [⇔]
→ Pseudobulbar palsy [⇔]

| XI | Spinal accessory | Motor | • Trapezius – shrug shoulders against resistance |
| | | | • Sternocleidomastoids – turn head against resistance |

		Conclusion	• Wash / gel hands, thank pt
			• Perform fundoscopy
			• Investigations: CT / MRI brain, formal hearing test

CRANIAL NERVES

Causes of specific cranial nerve palsies

- I Olfactory
  - Trauma
  - Frontal lobe tumour
  - Meningitis
- II Optic
  - Monocular blindness
    - MS
    - GCA
  - Bitemporal hemianopia
    - Pituitary adenoma
    - Internal carotid artery aneurysm
  - Homonymous hemianopia
    - Anything behind chiasm
    - Stroke / tumour / abscess
- III Oculomotor
  - Partial (pupil spared)
    - Diabetes*
  - Complete
    - PCA aneurysm
    - Raised ICP with tentorial herniation
- IV Trochlear
  - Single palsy rare
  - Usually due to orbit trauma
- V Trigeminal
  - Idiopathic (trigeminal neuralgia)
  - Acoustic neuroma
  - Herpes zoster
- VI Abducens
  - Skull # involving petrous temporal bone
  - Nasopharyngeal carcinoma
  - Raised ICP (false localising sign)

- VII Facial
  - LMN (forehead affected)
    - Bell's palsy
    - Malignant parotid tumour
    - Herpes zoster (Ramsay Hunt)
    - Sarcoid (often bilateral)
  - UMN (forehead spared)
    - Stroke / tumour
- VIII Vestibulocochlear
  - Excessive noise levels
  - Ménière's disease
  - Furosemide
  - Aminoglycoside antibiotics (gentamicin)
- IX / X / XII Bulbar [p73]
  - LMN (bulbar palsy)
    - MND
    - Diphtheria
    - Polio
    - Myasthenia gravis
    - Guillain–Barré syndrome
    - Syringobulbia
  - UMN (pseudobulbar palsy)
    - Motor neurone disease
    - Bilateral strokes
    - MS

*In diabetic oculomotor palsy the pial vessels perfusing parasympathetic fibres are unaffected by the diabetic microangiopathy, hence the pupil is spared (and the palsy 'partial')

NOTES

CRANIAL NERVES NOTES

Causes of grouped cranial nerve palsies

- Cerebellopontine angle tumour (acoustic neuroma or meningioma)
  - ○ Corneal reflex lost first (V)
  - ○ Then VII & VIII
  - ○ Then rest of V
  - ○ Sometimes IX & X
- Paget's disease of bone (bony impingement on nerves)
  - ○ V, VII & VIII
- Gradenigo's syndrome (complication of otitis media)
  - ○ V & VI
- Syringobulbia
  - ○ Bulbar palsy (IX, X & XII)
  - ○ VIII – vertigo & nystagmus
  - ○ V – facial pain / sensory loss
  - ○ VII sparing
  - ○ May have Horner's syndrome
  - ○ May have syringomyelia [p61]
- Cavernous sinus thrombosis
  - ○ III, IV & VI (VI most common)
  - ○ V – pain (especially ophthalmic division)
  - ○ Corneal reflex may be lost (V)
  - ○ Also headache, periorbital oedema, proptosis

Causes of *any* cranial nerve palsy

- Diabetes ('microangiopathy of the vasa nervorum')
- Stroke
- MS
- Tumour
- Sarcoid
- SLE
- Vasculitis

ΔΔ Ptosis

- Unilateral
  - ○ CN III palsy
  - ○ Horner's syndrome
  - ○ Congenital
- Bilateral
  - ○ Myasthenia gravis
  - ○ Myotonic dystrophy
  - ○ Congenital

Features of CN III palsy

- Eye deviated 'down and out'
- Ptosis
- Dilated pupil if complete*

Extra-ocular muscles
- CN III
  - ○ Superior rectus
  - ○ Inferior rectus
  - ○ Medial rectus
  - ○ Inferior oblique
- CN IV
  - ○ Superior oblique – 'SO4'
- CN VI
  - ○ Lateral rectus – 'LR6'

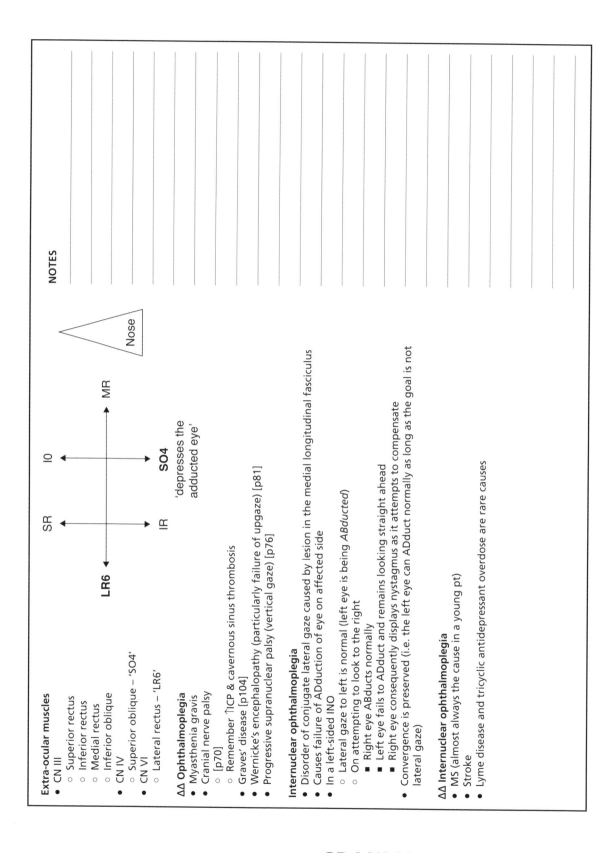

ΔΔ Ophthalmoplegia
- Myasthenia gravis
- Cranial nerve palsy
  - ○ [p70]
  - ○ Remember ↑ICP & cavernous sinus thrombosis
- Graves' disease [p104]
- Wernicke's encephalopathy (particularly failure of upgaze) [p81]
- Progressive supranuclear palsy (vertical gaze) [p76]

Internuclear ophthalmoplegia
- Disorder of conjugate lateral gaze caused by lesion in the medial longitudinal fasciculus
- Causes failure of ADduction of eye on affected side
- In a left-sided INO
  - ○ Lateral gaze to left is normal (left eye is being *ABducted*)
  - ○ On attempting to look to the right
    - ■ Right eye ABducts normally
    - ■ Left eye fails to ADduct and remains looking straight ahead
    - ■ Right eye consequently displays nystagmus as it attempts to compensate
- Convergence is preserved (i.e. the left eye can ADduct normally as long as the goal is not lateral gaze)

ΔΔ Internuclear ophthalmoplegia
- MS (almost always the cause in a young pt)
- Stroke
- Lyme disease and tricyclic antidepressant overdose are rare causes

CRANIAL NERVES NOTES

Interpretation of Rinne & Weber tests:

Rinne test	Weber test	Diagnosis
Air > bone (both ears)	Central	Normal
Bone > air (left ear)	Lateralises to left ear	Conductive hearing loss in left ear
Bone > air (left ear)*	Lateralises to right ear	Complete sensorineural deafness in left ear
Air > bone (both ears)	Lateralises to left ear	Sensorineural hearing loss in right ear

*In this interesting situation, during the Rinne test, sound is conducted via the skull across to the (normal) right ear when bone conduction is tested. Nothing is heard when air conduction is tested. Therefore bone is louder than air.

Features of bulbar & pseudobulbar palsies:

	Lesion	Aetiology	Tongue appearance (use to differentiate)	Other features
Bulbar palsy	LMN	• MND** • Diphtheria • Polio • Myasthenia gravis • Guillain-Barré syndrome • Syringobulbia	• Flaccid • Wasted • Fasciculating	• Drooling • Dysphonia • Tremulous lips
Pseudobulbar palsy	UMN	• MND** • Bilateral strokes (e.g. internal capsule) • MS	• Spastic • Contracted	• Drooling • Dysphonia • Emotional lability

** Note MND can cause either

NOTES

	Action / Examine for	ΔΔ / Potential findings / Extra information
Introduction	• Wash / gel hands • Introduce yourself, confirm pt, explain examination & gain consent • Position (ideally supine at 45° but the majority of the examination can be done seated)	

General inspection	• Poverty of facial expression
	  ○ 'Mask-like' face
	  ○ Loss of facial micro-movements
	• Flexed extrapyramidal posture
	  ○ Cannot lie flat (head held off pillow)
	  ○ 'Simian posture' on standing
	    ■ Stooped
	    ■ Hands held in front of groins
		→ 'Hands over hernias' position

Core features of parkinsonism (TRAP)

	Action / Examine for	ΔΔ / Potential findings / Extra information

Tremor	• Look for Parkinsonian tremor with hands resting on a pillow
	  ○ Coarse tremor (3–4 Hz)
	  ○ Pill-rolling quality
	• Ask pt to hold hands out in front of them, fingers spread
	  ○ Parkinsonian tremor should improve
	• Consider other causes of tremor
	  ○ Tremor which worsens with hands held up
	  ○ Titubation (no–no or yes–yes head movement)
	  ○ Flapping tremor – assess formally if you suspect this
		→ Hallmark of true resting tremor
		
		→ Postural tremor
		→ Essential tremor [↔]
		→ Hepatic / respiratory / renal failure

Rigidity	• "Let your arm go completely floppy" • Take hand in 'shaking hands' grip, supporting arm at elbow • Pronate / supinate to detect supinator catch • Flex / extend wrist • Flex / extend elbow • "Tap your knee with your other hand" – continue to flex / extend elbow • Repeat with other arm	→ 'Cogwheeling' in parkinsonism → Synkinesis – reinforces hypertonia
Akinesia	• Ask pt to touch thumb to each finger in turn, as quickly as possible • Hold hands out in front & pretend to play piano	→ 'Bradykinesia' is a more accurate description → Look for slowness in these movements

EXTRAPYRAMIDAL NEUROLOGY / TREMOR

Postural instability
- Ask pt to rise from chair, walk across room, turn & come back
- Look for parkinsonian features
  - Hesitancy
  - Shuffling gait
  - Loss of arm swing
  - Hurried steps
  - Festination
  - Retropulsion

→ Slow to rise from chair, move off & turn around
→ The 'marche à petit pas'

→ Speeding up inadvertently
→ Falling backwards as feet rush ahead

Other tests
- Glabellar tap
  - Ask pt to fix eyes on a point on the wall
  - "I am going to tap on your forehead"
  - Tap repeatedly between their eyes with your index finger
  - Look for failure of attenuation of the blink response
- Speech
  - Ask pt to state name & date of birth
  - Listen for slow, monotonous speech
- Writing
  - Ask pt to write name & address
  - Look for micrographia
  - May also highlight functional difficulty

→ In the normal individual blinking will stop after 2–3 taps

→ Small handwriting

Function
- Ask pt to make motion of turning a tap
- Undo then do up a button
- Handle some coins

Conclusion
- Wash / gel hands & thank pt
- "I would like to assess for evidence of a Parkinson plus syndrome"
  - Perform a full neurological examination
  - Check erect & supine BP
  - Assess eye movements

→ Multi-system atrophy
→ Shy–Drager syndrome
→ Progressive supranuclear palsy

EXTRAPYRAMIDAL NEUROLOGY / TREMOR

Core features of Parkinsonism (TRAP)
Use this to guide examination sequence
- **T**remor
- **R**igidity
- **A**kinesia (or more accurately bradykinesia)
- **P**ostural instability

Conditions with similar presentations to Parkinsonism
- Benign essential tremor
- Wilson's disease
  - Tremor
  - Dyskinesias
  - Psychiatric illlness
  - Hepatotoxicity
  - Kayser–Fleischer rings in eyes

Causes of Parkinsonism
- Idiopathic Parkinson's disease
- Drug-induced Parkinsonism
  - Lithium
  - Phenothiazine antipsychotics
  - Atypical antipsychotics (less so)
  - Metoclopramide
- Parkinson-plus syndrome
  - Shy–Drager syndrome (autonomic failure)
  - Multi-system atrophy (cerebellar and pyramidal features)
  - Progressive supranuclear palsy (ocular features, including failure of vertical gaze)
- Atherosclerotic pseudoparkinsonism (legs only, less tremor)
- Dementia pugilistica
  - Parkinsonism due to repeated head trauma associated with boxing (e.g. Muhammad Ali)

Long-term complications of L-dopa therapy
- Increasingly severe parkinsonism
- Autonomic neuropathy
- Dysphagia
- Dementia
- Dyskinesias
- Motor fluctuations (on–off / end of dose)

Treatments used in Parkinson's disease
- L-dopa
- Dopamine agonists
  - Ropinerole
  - Apomorphine SC infusion
  - (Bromocriptine – disused due to SEs)
- Anticholinergics
  - Procyclidine
  - Orphenadrine
- COMT inhibitors
  - Entacapone
- MAO-B inhibitors
  - Selegiline
- Glutamate antagonists
  - Amantadine

NOTES

You may be asked to examine purely tremor rather than the entire extrapyramidal system.
Remember that often tremors do not conform to textbook descriptions.

ΔΔ Tremor
- Resting: Parkinsonism
- Flapping: Hepatic failure (encephalopathy), respiratory failure (CO_2 retention), renal failure
- Intention: Cerebellar lesion
- Postural: Benign essential tremor, physiological tremor [see below]

	Benign essential tremor	Exaggerated physiological tremor
Aetiology	• Unknown • Genetic component likely (family history in 50%)	• Fever • Hyperthyroidism • Anxiety states • Medication-induced (e.g. β_2-agonists)
Other information	• Improvement with alcohol • Progressive	• Non-progressive
Examination	• Mild asymmetry common • Usually slower (4–7 Hz) • Titubation in 50% • Postural & action	• Usually symmetrical • Usually faster (8–12 Hz) • No titubation • Usually purely postural (abolished on action)
Management	• β-blockers • Gabapentin if contraindicated	• Treat / remove cause if possible • β-blockers (or gabapentin) sometimes needed

EXTRAPYRAMIDAL NEUROLOGY / TREMOR NOTES 77

	Action / Examine for	ΔΔ / Potential findings / Extra information
Introduction	• Wash / gel hands • Introduce yourself, confirm pt, explain examination & gain consent • Expose & position pt (ideally down to shorts/pants, supine at 45°)	→ Consider a chaperone
General inspection	• Bruising, scars • Symmetry, muscle wasting, fasciculation	→ Recurrent falls → LMN lesion [p60]

Head		
Nystagmus	• *"Keep your head still and follow my finger"* • Move finger up, down, left & right quickly to elicit nystagmus	→ Nystagmus may be cerebellar [↩]
Speech	• Ask pt to read something aloud • Ask pt to say 'baby hippopotamus'	→ Staccato speech → Slurring

Upper limbs		
Tone	• Assess as per upper limb neurological exam [p58]	→ Hypotonia
Power	• Assess as per upper limb neurological exam [p58]	→ Reduced power may cause apparent impairment of co-ordination even in the absence of a cerebellar lesion

Co-ordination	• Rebound test
	  ○ Ask pt to put arms out straight in front, palms down and close eyes
	  ○ *"Keep your arms in that position"*
	  ○ Push each arm down in turn ~10 cm then release it
	  ○ Watch for arm bouncing back up to beyond original position
	• Finger–nose test
	  ○ Ask pt to touch their nose with one index finger
	  ○ Place your index finger directly in front of them ~50 cm away
	  ○ Ask to cycle between nose and your finger
	  ○ Slowly move your finger away from the pt so that they must stretch arm fully to touch it
	• Hand slapping test
	  ○ Ask if left- or right-handed then demonstrate test
	  ○ For example, left hand out, palm up
	  ○ Rest right hand in left hand, palm up
	  ○ Turn right hand over in left hand, to palm down
	  ○ Alternate right hand between palm up and down
	  ○ Look for slowness and difficulty
		→ Overshoot = dysmetria
		
		→ Dysmetria, past-pointing
		→ Intention tremor (more likely to be seen at extent of arm stretch)
		
		→ Always more difficult on non-dominant side
		
		→ Dysdiadochokinesis

CEREBELLAR FUNCTION

Lower limbs

Tone	• Assess as per lower limb neurological exam [p62]	→ Hypotonia
Power	• Assess as per lower limb neurological exam [p62]	→ As above
Co-ordination	• Foot tapping ○ Ask pt to tap foot on floor as rapidly as possible ○ Look for slowness and difficulty	→ Dysdiadochokinesis
	• Heel–shin test ○ At first guide pt through sequence by moving foot for them ○ Heel onto knee ○ Slide heel down front of shin ○ Lift off, bring foot back up and onto knee ○ Ask pt to continue moving their foot in this cycle	→ Intention tremor, dysmetria

Posture / gait

Posture	• *"How stable are you when sitting or standing up?"*	
	• Assess stability sitting ○ Sit on side of bed ○ Ask to cross arms in front and sit still	→ Truncal ataxia
	• Assess stability standing (only if stable sitting) ○ Feet together, arms by sides	→ Truncal ataxia
	• Romberg's test ○ Stand pt up, feet together, facing you ○ Hover your hands above pt's shoulders ○ *"Now close your eyes. I will catch you if necessary."* ○ If pt suddenly becomes very unsteady – positive test ○ Steady pt's shoulders and instruct to open eyes	→ Sensory ataxia (i.e. non-cerebellar) → Without visual input and with impaired proprioception pt cannot maintain balance
Gait	• Ask pt to walk across room and back, look for features of cerebellar gait ○ Wide-based gait ○ Unsteadiness with lateral veering ○ Irregular steps • Ask to walk heel–toe	→ Very difficult if cerebellar lesion

Conclusion

Conclusion	• Wash / gel hands, thank pt & allow them to re-dress • *"I would like to complete a full neurological examination"* • Investigations: MRI for visualising posterior fossa

CEREBELLAR FUNCTION

Causes of cerebellar disease
- Stroke
- Tumour
- MS
- Congenital (e.g. Arnold–Chiari)
- Friedreich's ataxia
- Alcohol abuse
- Thiamine deficiency (e.g. Wernicke's encephalopathy)
- Anti-epileptic medication

Localising the cerebellar lesion
- This may be impossible clinically
- Lesions may involve both the vermis and hemispheres
- Central (vermis) lesion symptoms tend to cause:
  - Truncal ataxia sitting & standing
  - Poor heel–toe
  - Slurred staccato speech
- Cerebellar hemisphere lesion symptoms tend to cause:
  - *Ipsilateral* limb ataxia (dysmetria, intention tremor, dysdiadochokinesis)
  - Nystagmus
  - Unsteady gait, falling towards side of lesion when walking

ΔΔ Nystagmus
- Congenital
  (tends to cause pendular nystagmus most marked in neutral position)
- Brainstem problem (e.g. INO)
  - MS
  - Stroke
  - Tumour
- Cerebellar disease
  - See list above
  - Particularly MS
- Vestibular apparatus problem
  (nystagmus tends to be worse when looking away from side of lesion)
  - Labyrinthitis
  - Ménière's disease
  - CN VIII lesion

Classic signs of cerebellar lesion (DANISH)
- **D**ysdiadochokinesis
- **A**taxia (limb / trunk)
- **N**ystagmus
- **I**ntention tremor
- **S**peech (slurred, staccato)
- **H**ypotonia

Features of cerebellar limb ataxia
- Dysmetria
- Past-pointing
- Intention tremor
- Dysdiadochokinesis

NOTES

CEREBELLAR FUNCTION NOTES

ΔΔ Dysarthria

- Facial nerve palsy (CN VII) – look for facial weakness
- Bulbar palsy – look for flaccid, wasted, fasciculating tongue
  - ○ MND
  - ○ Guillain–Barré
  - ○ Syringobulbia
- Pseudobulbar palsy – look for spastic, contracted tongue
  - ○ MND
  - ○ MS
  - ○ Bilateral stroke (e.g. internal capsule)
- Myasthenia gravis
- Cerebellar disease [see above]

Wernicke's encephalopathy

- Due to thiamine (vitamin B_1) deficiency
- Usually related to alcohol abuse
- If untreated (with IV thiamine replacement) may progress to irreversible Korsakoff's psychosis
- Classical clinical triad
  1. Acute confusional state
  2. Ophthalmoplegia (especially upgaze)
  3. Ataxia (and other cerebellar signs)

NOTES

	Action / Examine for	ΔΔ / Potential findings / Extra information
Introduction	• Wash / gel hands • Introduce yourself, confirm pt, explain examination & gain consent • Expose & position pt (top off, supine at 45°)	→ Consider a chaperone
General inspection	• Central obesity • Peripheral muscle wasting	→ This combination results in the classical 'orange on matchsticks' appearance of Cushing's
Hands	• Reduced skin fold thickness	→ Skin may feel like tissue paper
Arms	• Bruising • "I would like to measure blood pressure" • Test shoulder ABduction power	→ Fragile blood vessels → Hypertension → Proximal myopathy
Face	• Moon facies • Acne • Plethora • Hirsutism	
Chest / back	• Gynaecomastia in male • Interscapular fat pad – 'buffalo hump' • Supraclavicular fat pads • Kyphosis	→ Vertebral wedge # due to osteoporosis
Abdomen	• Purple striae • Central obesity	
Legs	• Bruising • Test hip girdle strength – ask pt to stand from chair with arms crossed	→ Proximal myopathy

Conclusion	• Wash / gel hands, thank pt & allow to re-dress
	• "I would like to know if the pt has been on steroid therapy and, if not, consider performing tests to ascertain the aetiology of the Cushing's syndrome."
	• Further investigations
	   ○ Blood and urine glucose
	   ○ U+Es
	   ○ Bone scan
		→ [↺]
		
		→ Diabetes mellitus
		→ Hypokalaemia
		→ Osteoporosis

CUSHING'S SYNDROME

	Action / Examine for	ΔΔ / Potential findings / Extra information
Introduction	• Wash / gel hands • Introduce yourself, confirm pt, explain examination & gain consent • Position pt (supine at 45° or sitting)	
General inspection	• Height • General size	→ Pt with acromegaly may be very tall or may be of normal height with large features

Hands	• Size
	• Pinch skin to assess skin fold thickness
	• Median nerve exam
	  ○ Thenar eminence wasting
	  ○ Thumb ABduction
	  ○ Sensation in lateral index finger
	  ○ Tinel / Phalen tests
	• Feel palms
		→ May be very large
		→ May be increased
		→ Carpal tunnel syndrome [p54]
		
		→ Boggy, sweaty palms indicate active disease

Arms	• "I would now measure blood pressure" • Test shoulder ABduction power	→ Hypertension → Proximal myopathy
Neck	• JVP • Goitre	→ May be raised in cardiomyopathy → Due to ↑growth hormone (note pt will be euthyroid)

Face	• Prominent supraorbital ridges
	• Prognathism (best seen from side)
	• Big ears, nose and lips
	• Large tongue
	• "Show me your gums"
	  ○ Prognathism causing underbite
	  ○ Wide separation of teeth
		→ Enlarged, protruding mandible
		
		→ ΔΔ Amyloidosis

Eyes	• Visual fields	→ Bitemporal hemianopia (often remains after surgery)
Legs	• Test hip girdle strength – ask pt to stand from chair with arms crossed	→ Proximal myopathy

Conclusion	• Wash / gel hands & thank pt
	• "I would arrange an oral glucose tolerance test with growth hormone and IGF-1 measurement"
	• Perform full cardiovascular examination & 12-lead ECG
	• Further investigations
	  ○ Blood and urine glucose
	  ○ MRI
		→ Failure of GH suppression confirms diagnosis
		
		→ Hypertension & cardiomyopathy
		
		→ Diabetes mellitus
		→ Pituitary adenoma

ACROMEGALY

Cushing's syndrome

- Cardiovascular system
  - Hypertension
  - Fluid retention & overload
- Gastrointestinal system
  - Fatty liver
  - Pancreatitis
- Neurological system
  - Euphoria
  - Depression
  - Psychosis
  - Insomnia
- Locomotor system
  - Proximal myopathy
  - Osteoporosis
  - Vertebral wedge fractures
  - Avascular necrosis (e.g. femoral head)
- Immune system
  - Immunosuppression
- Endocrine system
  - Diabetes mellitus
- General cushingoid features
  - Central obesity
  - Muscle wasting in limbs
  - Thin skin
  - Bruising
  - Moon facies
  - Facial plethora
  - Acne
  - Hirsutism
  - Buffalo hump
  - Gynaecomastia
  - Purple abdominal striae

Causes of Cushing's syndrome

- High ACTH
  - Pituitary adenoma (Cushing's disease)
  - Ectopic ACTH (e.g. SCLC)
- Low ACTH
  - Adenoma of adrenal cortex
  - Carcinoma of adrenal cortex
  - Iatrogenic (corticosteroid therapy)

Common indications for long-term corticosteroid Rx

- Respiratory
  - Asthma
  - COPD
  - Pulmonary fibrosis
- Gastrointestinal
  - Inflammatory bowel disease
  - Autoimmune hepatitis
- Rheumatology
  - RA
  - SLE
  - Polymyalgia rheumatica
  - GCA
  - Vasculitis
  - Myositis
- Dermatology
  - Psoriasis
  - Severe eczema
  - Pemphigus & pemphigoid
- Transplant
- Replacement doses (should not cause Cushing's)
  - Addison's disease
  - Hypopituitarism

Investigation of non-iatrogenic Cushing's syndrome

1. Preliminary diagnosis
   - Overnight dexamethasone suppression test

   or
   - 24-hour urinary free cortisol
2. Confirm diagnosis
   - 48-hour dexamethasone suppression test
3. Localise lesion
   - Plasma ACTH
   - High dose dexamethasone suppression test (some response suggests Cushing's disease)
   - Imaging:
     - CT (chest / adrenals)
     - MRI (pituitary fossa)

NOTES

CUSHING'S SYNDROME NOTES

Treatment of acromegaly
- Trans-sphenoidal resection of tumour
- Bromocriptine / octreotide
  - Reduce growth hormone synthesis
  - Used in young adults due to high risk of infertility following surgery
  - May be used pre-operatively

ΔΔ Proximal myopathy
- Cushing's syndrome
- Acromegaly
- Hyperthyroidism
- Muscular dystrophy
- Polymyositis
- Dermatomyositis
- Myasthenia gravis
- Hypo / hyper K$^+$
- Hypo / hyper Ca^{2+}

NOTES

Action / Examine for	ΔΔ / Potential findings / Extra information
Introduction	
• Wash / gel hands	
• Introduce yourself, confirm pt, explain examination & gain consent	
• Expose & position pt (down to pants or shorts, supine at 45°)	→ Consider chaperone
• "Are you sore anywhere in your legs or feet?"	
Inspection	
• Colour	
○ Pallor	→ Ischaemia (especially acute)
○ Mottling	→ Acute ischaemia (unlikely in OSCE!)
○ Redness with dependency	→ Chronic ischaemia [↔]
○ Black	→ Tissue necrosis / gangrene
• Peripheral oedema	→ Venous disease [p139]
• Trophic changes	→ Chronic arterial disease
○ Pale skin	
○ Hair loss	
○ Onychogryphosis	→ Thickened, distorted nail
○ Fungal infections (skin / nails)	
• Guttering of superficial veins	→ Chronic arterial disease
• Ulcers	[↔ for arterial vs. venous]
○ Site	
○ Edge	
○ Exudate	
• Scars	→ Fem-pop bypass, fem-distal bypass
• Quickly look for abdominal scars	→ Aorto-bifemoral graft
Palpation	
• Temperature	→ Cold implies arterial insufficiency
○ Use back of hand	
○ Compare sides	
○ Use one of your hands only (i.e. *not* both hands at once)	
• Capillary refill time	→ Normally 1–2 sec
○ Increased	→ PVD / ischaemia
○ Reduced	→ Dependent blood pooling [↔]

LOWER LIMB ARTERIAL SYSTEM

Pulses	- Always move from proximal to distal
	- Assess rate, rhythm, character & symmetry
	- Move from side to side
	- Femoral
	   ○ Half-way between ASIS & pubic symphysis → *half way btwn ASIS & pubic symphysis · Mid-inguinal point - cf. mid point of inguinal ligament → half way btwn ASIS & pubic tubercle*
	   ○ Below inguinal ligament
	   ○ Demonstrate use of surface anatomy
	   ○ Auscultate for femoral bruits → *Femoral artery disease*
	- Popliteal
	   ○ Flex knee to 30°, ensure pt relaxed → *Often hard to feel – don't worry if you can't (and don't pretend you can!)*
	   ○ Grasp knee with both hands, thumbs in front, feel with fingers
	- Posterior tibial
	   ○ Behind medial maleolus
	- Dorsalis pedis
	   ○ Between bases of 1st & 2nd metatarsals

Special tests	- Buerger's test
	   ○ Lie pt flat
	   ○ Normal side first
	   ○ Slowly perform straight leg raise
	   ○ Look for 'guttering' of superficial veins
	   ○ Note point at which leg goes pale – angle between leg and the
	     horizontal at this point is 'Buerger's angle' → *Shallower angle = more severe PVD*
	- Quick version (if short of time)
	   ○ Lift leg straight up to ~70° hip flexion → *Check no hip pain first*
	   ○ Assess capillary refill time → *Increased in PVD* *Swing leg off bed – test for reactive hyperaemia*

Conclusion	- Wash / gel hands, thank pt & allow to re-dress
	- Measure BP
	- Measure ankle-brachial pressure index
	- Assess for risk factors for peripheral arterial disease
	   ○ Tar staining on hands
	   ○ Stigmata of hypercholesterolaemia
	- Further investigations: Doppler USS, MRA → [↥]

& Circⁿ for AAA

LOWER LIMB ARTERIAL SYSTEM

Beware the pt with one red foot and one pale foot (often with *rapid* CRT in the red foot)
- Easy to think the white foot is the ischaemic one
- In fact the whiter foot may be normal, with the red foot occurring due to dependent pooling of venous blood in a chronically ischaemic limb (the pt may have been sitting up in a chair prior to your arrival)
- Before commenting, feel the temperature of the feet and see what happens to the red foot when it is elevated from the bed – if ischaemic it will rapidly exsanguinate and become very pale

Causes of 'claudication' in presence of normal peripheral pulses
1. Neurogenic claudication (spinal stenosis [p48])
2. Anaemia
3. β-blockers

Critically ischaemic limb (6 Ps)
- Pain
- Pallor
- Pulseless
- Perishingly cold
- Paraesthesia
- Paralysis (best indicator of danger to limb)

ABPI measurements
>1	Normal
0.5–1	Intermittent claudication
0.3–0.5	Rest pain / critical limb ischaemia
<0.3	Gangrene + ulceration

Arterial supply to the lower limbs

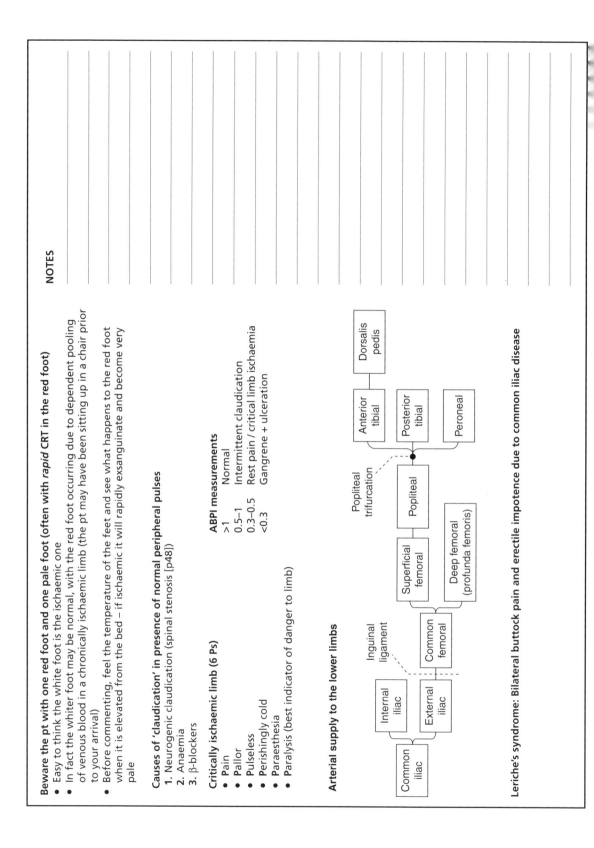

Leriche's syndrome: Bilateral buttock pain and erectile impotence due to common iliac disease

NOTES

	Venous ulcer	Arterial ulcer
History	• Varicose veins • DVTs	• Intermittent claudication • Rest pain
Classic sites	• Medial gaiter region of lower leg	• Feet / toes • Ankle (lateral maleolus)
Edges	• Sloped	• Punched-out
Exudate	• Lots	• Usually little
Pain	• Not severe unless associated with excessive oedema or infection	• Painful
Oedema	• Usually associated with limb oedema	• Oedema uncommon
Associated features	• Venous eczema • Haemosiderosis • Lipodermatosclerosis • Atrophie blanche	• Trophic changes _ hair loss, onychogryphosis . • Gangrene

Management	• Graduated compression dressing
	• Antibiotics for infection
		• Conservative
		• Endovascular revascularisation (angioplasty)
		• Surgical revascularisation (depends on sites of disease)
		   ○ Fem-pop bypass
		   ○ Fem-distal bypass
		   ○ Axillo-femoral bypass
		   ○ Aorto-bifemoral graft

NOTES

LOWER LIMB ARTERIAL SYSTEM NOTES

	Action / Examine for	ΔΔ / Potential findings / Extra information
Introduction	• Wash / gel hands • Introduce yourself, confirm pt, explain examination & gain consent • Expose & position pt (down to pants or shorts, standing) • *"Are you sore anywhere in your legs or feet?"*	→ Consider chaperone

Inspection	• Varicose veins
	  ○ Posterior lower leg
	  ○ Medial lower leg & thigh
	• Saphena varix
	• Blue-ish lump in groin apparent when standing
	• Signs of progressive chronic venous insufficiency
	  ○ Oedema
	  ○ Venous eczema
	  ○ Haemosiderosis
	    ■ Brown speckled discoloration
	    ■ 'Cayenne pepper petechiae'
	    ■ Especially medial gaiter area
	  ○ Lipodermatosclerosis
	    ■ Scarring of subcutaneous fat
	    ■ Skin tight and indurated
	    ■ May cause 'inverted champagne bottle' legs
	  ○ Atrophie blanche
	    ■ White scar-like areas ~~(from healed ulcers?)~~
	  ○ Ulceration
	    ■ Especially medial gaiter area
	
	progression →
		→ Short saphenous system
		→ Long saphenous system
		→ Dilated SFJ (2° incompetence)
		→ Usually disappears when supine
		
		→ [p139 for ΔΔ]
		
		→ Very common – extravasation of haemosiderin (a blood breakdown product) due to venous hypertension
		
		→ Disproportionately narrow ankles; also caused by CMT [p36]
		
		→ [p89 for features]

Palpation	• Skin texture for lipodermatosclerosis
	  ○ Hard
	  ○ 'Woody'
	• Calf tenderness
	• Varicose veins
	  ○ Tenderness
	  ○ Temperature (warmth)
	• Saphenofemoral incompetence
	  ○ Locate pubic tubercle
	  ○ Approximate position of SFJ is 2 cm inferior & lateral
	  ○ May be marked by presence of saphena varix ~~large varicosity on SFJ~~
	  ○ With fingers in this position (or on varix) ask pt to cough
	  ○ Feel for cough impulse – if present +ve test
		→ DVT
		→ Superficial phlebitis
		→ Superficial phlebitis
		
		↳ *transmitted pressure → of venous blood in SFJ*
		→ Exclude hernia which can also cause cough impulse in groin [p98]

Special tests

- Trendelenburg (tourniquet) test → Identifies level of venous incompetence *(only perform if can see varicose veins)*
  - Have pt lie flat
  - Perform straight leg raise & put leg on your shoulder
  - Expedite emptying of veins by stroking them towards groin
  - Once empty, apply tourniquet tightly in upper thigh
  - Have pt stand up
  - Look for varicosities filling for 10–15 sec then release tourniquet
  - 2 common outcomes
    - No filling on standing & rapid filling on release of tourniquet → Isolated sapheno-femoral junction incompetence
    - Slow filling on standing & rapid filling on release of tourniquet → Mixed sapheno-femoral junction and perforating vein incompetence

Conclusion

- Wash / gel hands, thank pt & allow to re-dress
- *"I would like to examine the lower limb arterial system and neurology"*
- Perform Perthes test → Ulcers may be multifactorial
- Further investigations: Doppler USS to identify sites of incompetence → Distinguish antegrade & retrograde flow in superficial varices

LOWER LIMB VENOUS SYSTEM

How to present your findings

In the common case of a patient with obvious varicose veins

- There are varicose veins in the distribution of the [long / short / both] saphenous systems
- There [is / is no] saphena varix
- Trendelenburg test suggests [sapheno-femoral / mixed sapheno-femoral and perforator] incompetence
- There [are / are no] associated features of chronic venous insufficiency
- There [is / is no] evidence of superficial thrombophlebitis

Example: The pt has varicose veins of both legs in the distribution of the long saphenous systems. There are saphena varices bilaterally with positive cough impulses. The Trendelenburg test indicates isolated sapheno-femoral incompetence. There are associated features of chronic venous insufficiency, namely oedema, haemosiderosis and lipodermatosclerosis. There is no evidence of superficial thrombophlebitis.

Varicose veins

- Occur as a result of valvular incompetence
  - Structural predisposition (familial tendency)
- Factors that ↑ venous pressure: prolonged standing, obesity, pregnancy
- Sites of incompetence
  - Sapheno-femoral junction (SFJ) – typically causes long saphenous vein (LSV) varices
  - Sapheno-popliteal junction (SPJ) – typically causes short saphenous vein (SSV) varices
  - Perforating veins linking deep veins and saphenous systems
- Often associated with signs of chronic venous insufficiency [see over]

Management of varicose veins

- Conservative
  - Elastic support hose
  - Weight loss
  - Regular exercise
  - Avoid prolonged standing
- Injection sclerotherapy
  - Suitable for small varices below knee due to incompetence of local perforators
  - Not satisfactory for varices associated with SFJ incompetence (recurrence inevitable)

- Surgery
  - SFJ incompetence & LSV varices
    - SFJ ligated (a so-called 'high tie')
    - LSV usually stripped from knee to groin (reduced chance of recurrence) stab avulsions of remaining varices
  - SPJ incompetence & SSV varices
    - SPJ ligated (SSV not stripped due to risk of damaging sural nerve)
    - Stab avulsions of remaining varices
- Newer techniques
  - Ultrasound-guided foam sclerotherapy
  - Radiofrequency or laser obliteration of LSV / SSV

LOWER LIMB VENOUS SYSTEM NOTES

Causes of chronic venous insufficiency
1. Valvular incompetence of deep veins (90%)
   ○ Primary (aetiology same as for varicose veins)
   ○ Secondary (damaged by DVT)
2. Obstruction of deep veins by DVT (10%)

Chronic venous insufficiency 2° DVT = 'post-thrombotic syndrome'

Superficial thrombophlebitis
- Inflammation and thrombosis almost invariably occurring in varicose veins
- Redness and tenderness follow line of vein
- Thrombosis may spread to deep system and cause DVT
- Management
  ○ Analgesia
  ○ NSAIDs
  ○ Support stockings
  ○ Active exercise
- Underlying vein usually removed as recurrence is common
- Propagation towards deep veins is an indication for IV heparin

NOTES

LOWER LIMB VENOUS SYSTEM NOTES

General Examination of a Lump

This sequence can be used to assess any lump or swelling. Tailored examination of lumps in specific areas is covered in the subsequent sections: groin herniae, ventral herniae, neck lump, breast lump, scrotal swelling.

	Action / Examine for	ΔΔ / Potential findings / Extra information
Introduction	• Wash / gel hands • Introduce yourself, confirm pt, explain examination & gain consent • *"Where have you noticed the lump? Are there any more anywhere?"* • Expose relevant areas & position pt so comfortable	→ Consider chaperone depending on lump location

Inspection	• Site
	• Relationship to surrounding anatomical structures
	• General idea of size and shape
	• Overlying skin
	   ○ Colour
	   ○ Punctum
	   ○ Discharge
		→ Better assessed by palpation
		
		→ Erythema
		→ Typical of sebaceous cyst
		→ Abscess

Palpation of lump	• *"Tell me if you feel any discomfort"*
	• Put your fingers on the centre of the lump
	   ○ Surface
	   ○ Consistency
	   ○ Heat
	   ○ Tenderness
	• Move to the borders
	   ○ Shape
	   ○ Size
	   ○ Edge
	• Assess fluctuance
	   ○ 'Bounce' lump between your two index fingers
	• Attachment to skin
	   ○ Try to slide skin over the lump
	• Attachment to other structures
	   ○ Ask pt to assume a position that contracts the underlying musculature – try to move lump
	   ○ If suspicious of a ganglion, ask pt to move joint that involves that particular tendon & feel if lump moves too
	• Feel for special characteristics
	   ○ Thrill
	   ○ Pulsation
	• Transilluminate with pen torch
		→ Watch pt's face for evidence of discomfort
		
		→ Smooth, irregular, craggy
		→ Hard, firm, rubbery, soft
		→ Inflammation
		→ Inflammation
		
		→ Circular, oblong, 'pear-shaped', etc.
		→ Estimate in cm
		→ Well-defined, indistinct, irregular
		
		→ Lipomas are fluctuant
		
		→ Impossible if intradermal [⇨]
		
		→ Attachment to musculature is suspicious of malignancy
		→ Ganglion will move with tendon of origin
		
		→ AV fistula
		→ Aneurysm
		→ Cystic swelling

GENERAL LUMPS

	Action / Examine for	ΔΔ / Potential findings / Extra information

Palpation of nodes	• Palpate regional lymph nodes, especially if suspicion of malignancy
	  ○ Head & neck [p137 for technique]
	  ○ Axillary
	  ○ Groin	

Auscultation	• If palpable thrill or pulsation	→ Bruit in AV fistula

Conclusion	• Wash / gel hands, thank pt & allow to re-dress
	• If not done: "I would like to assess for regional lymphadenopathy"
	• "I would enquire about any changes which might raise suspicion of a malignant lump"
	  ○ Increasing size
	  ○ Changing surface / consistency / edge
	  ○ Development of associated pain
	• Investigations: imaging, biopsy
		→ Do not mention malignancy within earshot of pt if they have not been counselled about a possible cancer diagnosis
		
		→ May be due to local invasion

Examination of a Skin Lesion

	Action / Examine for	ΔΔ / Potential findings / Extra information
Introduction	• Wash / gel hands • Introduce yourself, confirm pt, explain examination & gain consent • "Have you noticed any abnormalities of your skin? Where?" • Expose relevant areas & position pt so comfortable	→ Consider chaperone depending on location of skin lesion
Inspection	• Site or distribution if multiple lesions • Size • Shape • Border • Colour • Discharge	→ Single lesion / rash → Regular, irregular, 'rolled' (BCC) → Erythema
Palpation	• Feel if elevated above surrounding skin • Tenderness • Heat	→ Macule (flat) / papule (elevated) → Inflammation → Inflammation
Conclusion	• Wash / gel hands, thank pt & allow to re-dress • "I would like to assess for regional lymphadenopathy then examine the rest of the pt's skin." • If malignancy suspected: "I would like to perform a full systematic examination to look for evidence of metastatic disease." • Investigations: bloods, biopsy, serial photographs	→ Do not mention malignancy within earshot of pt if they have not been counselled about a possible cancer diagnosis

Intradermal lumps (impossible to slide skin over)
- Sebaceous cyst
- Abscess
- Dermoid cyst
- Granuloma

Signs of inflammation
- Calor (heat)
- Dolor (pain)
- Rubor (erythema)
- Tumor (swelling)
- Loss of function

Subcutaneous lumps (skin can slide over)
- Lipoma
- Ganglion
- Neurofibroma
- Lymph node [p136]

NOTES

_____

_____

_____

_____

_____

Common benign lumps

	Lipoma	Sebaceous cyst	Ganglion
Description	Benign fatty tumour	Epidermal proliferation within dermis	Degenerative cyst from synovum of joint / tendon
Common sites	Anywhere fat can expand (*not* scalp or palms)	Anywhere on body (most common on trunk, neck, face & scalp)	Dorsum of hand / wrist Dorsal foot
Depth	Subcutaneous	Intradermal	Subcutaneous
Other features	Smooth Imprecise margins Fluctuant	Central punctum	Moves with tendon May transilluminate
Complications	Symptoms 2° pressure effects Malignant change (*very rare*)	Infection common	Rare
Management	Conservative Excision for cosmetic reasons or local pressure effects	Incision & drainage if infected Occasionally antibiotics needed Non-infected cysts can be 'shelled out' under local anaesthesia	Conservative (50% disappear) Aspiration Excision 'Blow from a Bible' (not advised!)

GENERAL LUMPS NOTES

Common skin lesions

- Melanocytic naevus (mole)
- Urticaria
- Eczema
- Ulcers [see below]
- Spider naevi
- Campbell de Morgan spots
- Striae (e.g. Cushing's syndrome)
- Skin tags
- Psoriasis
- Seborrhoeic keratosis
- Erythema nodosum
- Tumour
  - Melanoma
  - Squamous cell carcinoma
  - Basal cell carcinoma
- Neurofibromatosis (common in OSCEs!)
  - Neurofibromata
  - Café au lait spots

ΔΔ Erythema nodosum
Painful, purple, raised lesions on shins

- Idiopathic (up to 55% of cases)
- Sarcoidosis (30–40% of cases)
- Infection
  - *Streptococci*
  - TB
- IBD
- Drugs
  - OCP
  - Sulphonamides
- Malignancy
  - Lymphoma
  - Leukaemia
- Pregnancy

Neurofibromatosis

- Genetic disorder
- 2 variants (Type 1 & Type 2)
- Both types autosomal dominant
- Type 1 = von Recklinghausen's disease
  (this neurofibroma **CATCHES** on my clothes)
  - **C**afé au lait patches (>6 is diagnostic)
  - **A**xillary freckling
  - **T**umours of nervous system
  - **C**utaneous neurofibromata
  - **H**ypertension
  - **E**ye features (Lisch nodules)
  - **S**coliosis
- Type 2
  - Bilateral acoustic neuromas (key feature)
  - Other tumours of nervous system
  - Fewer cutaneous features

ΔΔ Ulcer by type of edge

- Sloping   Venous
- Punched-out Arterial   } [p89]
- Undermined TB, pressure necrosis
- Rolling   Basal cell carcinoma
- Everted   Squamous cell carcinoma

Warning signs of a melanoma (ABCDE)

- **A**symmetry
- **B**order irregularity
- **C**olour variation
- **D**iameter (>6 mm or increasing)
- **E**levation

NOTES

GROIN HERNIA

	Action / Examine for	ΔΔ / Potential findings / Extra information

Introduction	• Wash / gel hands
	• Introduce yourself, confirm pt, explain examination & gain consent
	• Expose pt (fully from waist down)
	• Ensure a chaperone is present
	• Position: Dependent on scenario
	   ○ If pt already supine & swelling obvious, examine supine
	   ○ If pt already supine & swelling not obvious, examine standing
	   ○ If pt already standing, examine standing
	• *"Can you show me where you have you noticed the abnormality?"*
	• *"Is it painful?"*
		→ Ensure privacy
		
		→ Herniae become more apparent on standing due to increased intra-abdominal pressure

Inspection	• Look for swellings on *both* sides • Scars (look carefully in groin creases) • *"Give me a loud cough"* – look for visible cough impulse	→ Previous surgical repair

Palpation	• Get down on one knee, keep checking pt's face
	• *"Let me know if you feel any discomfort"*
	• Start with quick feel of 'normal' side (if there is one)
	   ○ Palpable swelling
	   ○ Cough impulse
	• Move onto affected side
	   ○ Size of swelling
	   ○ Tension / heat / tenderness
	   ○ Try to locate lower extent of swelling
	   ○ Cough impulse
	• Locate pubic tubercle
	   ○ Hernia above tubercle = inguinal
	   ○ Hernia below tubercle = femoral
	• Palpate scrotum if ♂
	   ○ Extension of groin swelling
	   ○ Try to 'get above' any scrotal swelling
		→ May be a smaller, un-noticed hernia
		
		→ Strangulation
		→ If impossible may extend into scrotum in ♂
		→ If absent either incarcerated hernia or not a hernia at all (lymph node, cyst, lipoma, saphena varix)
		
		→ Usually indirect inguinal hernia
		→ If possible, swelling is not a hernia

Reduction	• Establish whether reducible
	   ○ Ask pt to reduce – *"Can you push the lump back inside?"*
	   ○ If unable, gently try to reduce yourself (with permission)
	   ○ If still unable and pt standing, try supine
	• Establish relationship to deep inguinal ring (if reducible)
	   ○ Reduce hernia
	   ○ Locate deep ring (half way between ASIS & pubic tubercle)
	   ○ Occlude deep ring with 2 fingers (and hernia still reduced)
	   ○ Ask pt to cough
	   ○ Does hernia reappear on coughing despite pressure on deep ring?
		→ Irreducible = incarcerated [↔]
		
		→ The midpoint of the inguinal ligament
		
		→ Reappears = direct. Held by pressure = indirect

Auscultation

- Auscultate over lump for bowel sounds → Hernia contents: bowel or omentum

Conclusion

- Wash / gel hands, thank pt & allow to re-dress
- If not done: "*I would like to examine the contralateral groin*"
- If examined supine: "*I would like to examine the groins with the pt standing to check for a small hernia on the contralateral side*"
- "*I would like to perform a full abdominal exam, in particular looking for a cause of raised intra-abdominal pressure*" → Hepatomegaly, splenomegaly, APKD, bladder distension, ascites, etc.
- Transillumination of any scrotal mass → Exclude a cystic scrotal swelling

GROIN HERNIA

Definition of a hernia: The protrusion of whole or part of a viscus through an opening in the wall of its containing cavity into a place where it is not normally found.

Features of groin hernias

	Indirect inguinal	Direct inguinal	Femoral
Route of herniation (*Fig. 24*)	Through internal inguinal ring, down inguinal canal and out of external ring	Through weak point in posterior wall of inguinal canal (Hesselbach's triangle*)	Through femoral canal underneath inguinal ligament
Relationship to pubic tubercle	Superior	Superior	Inferior
Extension into scrotum	Common	Rare	Impossible
Size	Can be very large	Moderate	Normally 3–5 cm
Reducible	Usually	Almost always	Rare (usually incarcerated with absent cough impulse)
Held by pressure on deep ring	✓	✗	✗
Complications	Low risk of incarceration and complication	Moderate risk of incarceration and complication	Usually incarcerated with high risk of strangulation
Management	Usually repaired as it is impossible to be 100% sure hernia is indirect on basis of clinical examination alone	Surgical repair	Urgent surgical repair

*Borders of Hesselbach's triangle
- Inferior epigastric artery
- Inguinal ligament
- Linea semilunaris (lateral border of rectus muscle)

Types of surgical hernia repair
- Open mesh repair (Lichtenstein)
- Open suture repair (Babinski / Shouldice)
- Laparoscopic
  ○ TEP (total extraperitoneal procedure)
  ○ TAP (trans-abdominal procedure)

Risk factors for developing a hernia
- Family history
- Weakness of abdominal musculature
  ○ Increasing age (especially direct)
  ○ Surgery (incisional hernia)
- Increased intra-abdominal pressure
  ○ Obesity
  ○ Pregnancy
  ○ Other organomegaly
  ○ COPD / chronic cough
  ○ Prostatism
  ○ Constipation
  ○ Heavy lifting

NOTES

GROIN HERNIA NOTES

Complications of a hernia:

Incarceration (irreducible)
→ 1. Obstruction (clinically: colic, constipation, vomiting, distension)
→ 2. Strangulation → ischaemia → necrosis → peritonitis

Richter's hernia
- Only part of the bowel wall herniates, allowing strangulation without obstruction
- More common in femoral hernia (narrower orifice)

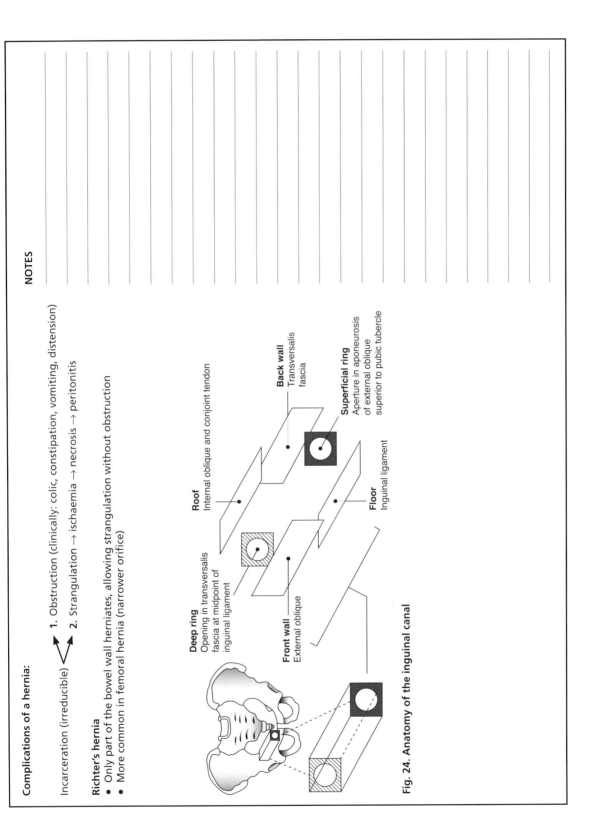

Deep ring
Opening in transversalis fascia at midpoint of inguinal ligament

Front wall
External oblique

Roof
Internal oblique and conjoint tendon

Back wall
Transversalis fascia

Floor
Inguinal ligament

Superficial ring
Aperture in aponeurosis of external oblique superior to pubic tubercle

Fig. 24. Anatomy of the inguinal canal

NOTES

Action / Examine for	ΔΔ / Potential findings / Extra information
Introduction	
• Wash / gel hands • Introduce yourself, confirm pt, explain examination & gain consent • Expose pt (entire neck)	→ Unbutton / remove top to see base of neck
End of bed	
• Thin, fidgety, tremulous, sweaty, flushed, restless • Fat, warmly dressed, hair loss, dry skin, deep voice	→ Hyperthyroid → Hypothyroid
Thyroid / Neck lump	
Inspection	

• *"Where is the area of concern?"*
• Look from front & sides
• Define location: midline, anterior / posterior triangle
• Swallowing
  ○ Ask pt to take sip of water and hold it in mouth
  ○ Instruct to swallow as you look from front
  ○ Repeat looking from side
• Stick out tongue
	→ Narrows the ΔΔ [↔]
	→ Thyroid moves upwards
	
	→ Thyroglossal cyst moves upwards

Palpation of neck lump	

• *"Have you any pain in your neck?"*
• Stand behind pt, use both hands to examine
  ○ Start in centre of lump, move out to edges
  ○ Size / shape / symmetry
  ○ Surface
  ○ Consistency
  ○ Edge
  ○ Fluctuance
  ○ Pulsation
• Specific to thyroid swelling
  ○ Diffuse enlargement or single nodule?
  ○ If diffuse, is it smooth or multinodular?
  ○ Lower extent – can you get below thyroid?
• Palpate from behind whilst pt swallows water
• Attempt to transilluminate lump
	→ Goitre [↔]
	  ○ Graves': soft, smooth, symmetrical
	  ○ MNG: firm, usually nodular, often asymmetrical (dominant nodule)
	
	→ Well defined, indistinct, irregular
	→ Lipoma
	→ Carotid body tumour
	
	→ If impossible goitre may extend retrosternally
	→ Thyroid moves on swallowing
	→ Neck cyst: thyroglossal, branchial, cystic hygroma

Palpation of nodes	
• Always perform this • Palpate systematically standing behind pt [p137]	
Percussion	
• Percuss sternum from xiphisternum up to suprasternal notch	→ Retrosternal goitre may cause dull percussion note
Auscultation	
• Both sides of lump (ask pt to hold breath)	→ Bruit is virtually diagnostic of Graves'
Special tests	

• Pemberton's test (if large goitre)
  ○ Slowly raise both arms above head
  ○ Watch for facial plethora
  ○ *"Take a deep breath in"* – listen for stridor
	→ Thoracic inlet obstruction due to a large retrosternal goitre
	→ Obstructed venous return from head
	→ Tracheal compression

THYROID / NECK LUMP / THYROID STATUS

Thyroid status (assess in any pt with goitre or thyroid symptoms)

		Hyperthyroid	Hypothyroid
Hands & wrist	Acropachy (clubbing)	Graves' [p138 for ΔΔ]	
	Palms	Hot, sweaty →	Cold, dry
	Palmar erythema	Yes	
	Paper (put on top of hands to detect fine tremor)	Yes	
	Pulse	Tachycardia ± AF	Bradycardia
Face	Facial appearance	Flushed	'Peaches & cream'
	Hair & eyebrows		Thin, brittle
	Eyes	[↔]	
	○ Exophthalmos	Graves'	
	○ Eyelids	Lid retraction	May be puffy
	Eye movements		
	○ "Follow my finger; tell me if you see double"		
	○ Move in 'H' pattern		
	○ Look for obvious ophthalmoplegia (esp. upgaze)	Graves'	
	Lid lag	Yes	
	○ Stand to side of pt		
	○ "Follow my finger, keep your head still"		
	○ Move finger upwards so you see lids retract		
	○ Quickly move finger downwards – look for delay in lids descending		
Limbs	Knee & biceps reflexes	Brisk	Slow-relaxing
	Carpal tunnel syndrome		Yes [p56]
	○ Median nerve power / sensation		
	○ Tinel / Phalen tests		
	Proximal myopathy	Yes	
	○ Shoulder ABduction		
	○ Stand up from chair with arms crossed (hip girdle strength)		
	Oedema	Grave's	
	○ Pre-tibial myxoedema		Yes
	○ Generalised non-pitting peripheral oedema		
Conclusion	• Wash / gel hands & thank pt		
	• If not done: "*I would like to assess thyroid status*"		
	• Investigations: TFTs, USS, FNA		

THYROID / NECK LUMP / THYROID STATUS

ΔΔ Neck lump

- Midline
  - ○ Goitre
  - ○ Thyroglossal cyst
- Anterior triangle
  - ○ Branchial cyst – under the top of SCM
  - ○ Carotid body tumour
  - ○ Lymph node [p137]
- Posterior triangle
  - ○ Cystic hygroma (above clavicle)
  - ○ Lymph node
- Anywhere
  - ○ Sebaceous cyst
  - ○ Lipoma [p96]

ΔΔ Goitre

- Multinodular goitre
- Graves' disease
- Solitary nodule (adenoma / carcinoma)
- Hashimoto's thyroiditis
- Subacute thyroiditis

ΔΔ Hypothyroidism

- Autoimmune
  - ○ Primary atrophic thyroiditis (no goitre)
  - ○ Hashimoto's initially
- Acquired
  - ○ Iodine deficiency (no. 1 cause worldwide)
  - ○ Subacute thyroiditis
  - ○ Iatrogenic
    - Surgery
    - Radioiodine
    - Carbimazole
    - Lithium
    - Amiodarone
- Secondary
  - ○ Panhypopituitarism (very rare)

Multinodular goitre (MNG)

- Most common large goitre
- Rarely can be smooth rather than multinodular to feel
- Pt usually euthyroid = non-toxic MNG
- Hyperthyroid = toxic MNG
- Indications for surgery in non-toxic MNG
  - ○ Cosmetic reasons
  - ○ Local compression effect

Graves' disease

- Classic features
  - ○ Goitre
  - ○ Thyrotoxicosis
  - ○ Eye disease (50%)
    - Exophthalmos
    - Ophthalmoplegia } Unique to Graves'
  - ○ Pretibial myxoedema
  - ○ Thyroid acropachy
- Factors differentiating from toxic MNG
  - ○ Smooth goitre (MNG rarely smooth)
  - ○ Graves'-unique features as above
  - ○ TSH-receptor antibodies
- Indications for surgery
  - ○ Cosmetic reasons
  - ○ Local compression effect
  - ○ Failed medical Rx
  - ○ Intolerant of medication

A note on thyroid eye signs

- Any cause of hyperthyroidism
  - ○ Lid retraction
  - ○ Lid lag
- Specific to Graves' disease
  - ○ Exophthalmos
  - ○ Ophthalmoplegia

ΔΔ Hyperthyroidism
- Graves'
- Toxic MNG   } 90%
- Toxic nodule (usually adenoma)
- Thyroiditis in the initial phase
  - Hashimoto's
  - Post-partum
  - Subacute
- Secondary (rare)
  - TSHoma
  - Hydatidiform mole
  - Choriocarcinoma

ΔΔ Parotid swelling
- Bilateral
  - Viral / bacterial parotitis
  - TB
  - Alcohol
  - Pleomorphic adenoma
  - Sjögren's
  - Sarcoidosis
- Unilateral
  - Duct blockage
  - Unilateral pleomorphic adenoma

Hyperthyroidism Rx
- Medical
  - Symptomatic control: β-blockers
  - Anti-thyroid therapy: carbimazole
- Radioiodine
- Surgical (cosmetic, compression, malignancy)
  - Total thyroidectomy
  - Subtotal thyroidectomy

Contraindications to radioiodine
- Pregnancy / breast feeding
- Young children at home
- Incontinent (eliminated in urine)

Complications of thyroidectomy
- Early
  - Anaesthetic / haemorrhage / infection
  - Damage to surrounding structures
    - Recurrent laryngeal nerve
    - Trachea
    - Oesophagus
    - Neck musculature
  - Transient hypoparathyroidism
- Late
  - Hypoparathyroidism
  - Recurrent hyperthyroidism
  - Hypothyroidism

NOTES

	Action / Examine for	ΔΔ / Potential findings / Extra information
Introduction	• Wash / gel hands, put on non-sterile gloves • Introduce yourself, confirm pt, explain examination & obtain consent • Expose pt (xiphisternum to pubic symphysis) • Position pt (lie flat with 1 pillow) • *"Do you have any pain in your tummy?"* • *"Have you had any problems with your stoma?"*	→ Consider chaperone

Inspection	• Site
	• Number of lumens
	• Spout
	• Effluent – *feel* the bag
	  ○ Hard stool
	  ○ Soft stool
	  ○ Urine
	• Surrounding skin quality
	• Complications
		[↬ for features of stoma types]
		
		Inflammation / excoriation
		[↬]

Auscultation	• Bowel sounds – just below umbilicus	→ Obstruction is a possible complication
Conclusion	• Wash / gel hands, thank pt & allow to re-dress • Stoma output chart • *"I would like to complete a full gastrointestinal & genitourinal examination"*	→ High or low output → As appropriate

106

STOMA

	Action / Examine for	ΔΔ / Potential findings / Extra information
Introduction	<ul><li>Wash / gel hands</li><li>Introduce yourself, confirm pt, explain examination & obtain consent</li><li>Expose pt (xiphisternum to pubic symphysis)</li><li>Position pt (standing or supine depending on situation – p98)</li><li>"Where have you noticed the abnormality? Is it painful?"</li></ul>	→ Consider chaperone
Inspection	<ul><li>Scars</li><li>"Give me a loud cough" – look for visible cough impulse</li><li>Ask pt to lift head off bed<ul><li>○ Accentuates hernia (especially incisional)</li><li>○ Rectus divarication</li></ul></li></ul>	→ Incisional hernia → Increases intra-abdominal pressure → Weakness of linea alba (common) [⇌]
Palpation	<ul><li>"Let me know if you feel any discomfort"<ul><li>○ Size of swelling</li><li>○ Tension / temperature / tenderness</li><li>○ Cough impulse</li></ul></li></ul>	→ Strangulation → Absent = incarcerated / not a hernia
Reduction	<ul><li>Establish whether reducible<ul><li>○ Ask pt to reduce – " Can you push that lump back inside for me?"</li><li>○ If unable, gently try to reduce yourself (with permission)</li><li>○ If still unable and pt standing, try supine</li></ul></li></ul>	→ Irreducible = incarcerated
Auscultation	<ul><li>Auscultate over lump for bowel sounds</li></ul>	→ Hernia contents: bowel or omentum
Conclusion	<ul><li>Wash / gel hands, thank pt & allow to re-dress</li><li>If examined supine: "I would now like to examine the patient standing"</li><li>"I would like to perform a full abdominal exam, in particular looking for a cause of raised intra-abdominal pressure"</li><li>Investigations: abdominal wall USS, CT abdomen</li></ul>	→ Hepatomegaly, splenomegaly, APKD, bladder distension, ascites, etc.

VENTRAL HERNIA

Examination of a Stoma

How to present your findings (stoma)

To present your findings, run through the following order

1. Site
2. Number of lumens
3. Spout / flush with skin
4. Nature of effluent
5. State of surrounding skin
6. Evidence of complication
7. Likely type of stoma
8. Possible procedure / underlying pathology

Example: The pt has a stoma in the left iliac fossa with a single lumen, which is flush with the skin and producing hard faeces. The surrounding skin is intact and shows no evidence of inflammation. There is no evidence of any other stoma complication. This is most likely an end-colostomy which usually follows abdomino-perineal resection or Hartmann's procedure. The indication may have been a rectal malignancy. I would like to go on and perform a full gastrointestinal examination, and inquire as to whether the pt still has an anus [see below].

Features of different stoma types

	Site	Lumens	Spout	Effluent	Possible procedure
End colostomy*	Usually left	1	✗	Hard stool	→ Abdomino-perineal (AP) resection → Hartmann's procedure with rectum oversewn
End ileostomy	Usually right	1	✓	Soft or liquid stool	→ Panproctocolectomy (e.g. UC, FAP) → Emergency subtotal colectomy

Loop ileostomy
(usually temporary)
	Usually right	2 (joined)	✓	Soft or liquid stool	→ To defunction
					  ○ Obstruction (e.g. malignancy)
					  ○ Anus (e.g. Crohn's)
					  ○ Newly formed anastamosis

Loop colostomy (usually temporary)	Upper abdomen	2 (joined)	✗	Hard stool	→ As above
End colostomy & mucous fistula	Usually left	2 (separate)	✗	Hard stool	→ Hartmann's procedure with rectum brought to skin
Urostomy	Either side	1	✓	Urine	→ Cystectomy (e.g. malignancy)

STOMA NOTES

*If pt has an end-colostomy
- Ask: *"Do you mind telling me if you still have a back passage following your operation?"*
- No = AP resection for low rectal tumour
- Yes = Hartmann's procedure for higher tumour

Ideal site for a stoma
- Healthy skin
- Away from umbilicus & belt line
- Avoiding
  - Bony prominences
  - Scars
  - Skin creases

Stoma complications
- Haemorrhage
- Necrosis
- Prolapse
- Retraction
- Obstruction
- Peristomal skin inflammation
- Parastomal hernia
- High output

Examination of a Ventral Hernia

Definition of a hernia: The protrusion of whole or part of a viscus through an opening in the wall of its containing cavity into a place where it is not normally found.

	Features	Surgical indications
Para-umbilical (acquired)	• Through linea alba, usually above umbilicus (rarely below) • Often irreducible	→ Always repaired (high risk of incarceration)
True umbilical (congenital)	• Through umbilicus • Usually resolve spontaneously in early life	→ Indicated if persists beyond 5 years of age
Epigastric	• Through linea alba in epigastrium • More common in thin individuals • 20% multiple, 80% just off midline	→ Usually repaired (moderate risk of incarceration)
Spigelian	• Through linea semilunaris at outer border of rectus sheath	→ Always repaired (high risk)
Incisional	• Can occur anywhere but especially midline surgery • Usually enlarge progressively & become cosmetic problem	→ Incarceration → Cosmetic issues
Rectus divarication	• Not actually a hernia • Weakness of linea alba leads to bulge in epigastrium • Sometimes associated with paraumbilical & epigastric hernias	→ Cosmetic issues

	Action / Examine for	ΔΔ / Potential findings / Extra information

Introduction	• Wash / gel hands & put on non-sterile gloves
	• Introduce yourself, confirm pt, explain examination & gain consent
	• In particular, explain
	  ○ The examination may be uncomfortable
	  ○ You will proceed slowly and gently
	  ○ The patient can stop you at any time
	• Ensure a chaperone is present
	• Ask if patient would like to go to the toilet before starting
	• Expose & position pt (bare below umbilicus, supine, hips & knees flexed, heels together, thighs abducted)
		→ Allow pt time & privacy to get undressed & lie supine on couch with sheet over their hips before you enter room / cubicle and position them

Inspection	• Ensure good lighting, systematically examine the entire vulva
	  ○ PV discharge or bleeding
	  ○ Atrophic change
	  ○ Ulcers
	  ○ Abnormal hair distribution
	  ○ Lumps
	• Part the labia and ask the patient to cough or 'bear down'
		→ Mons pubis – labia majora – labia minora – introitus – urethra – clitoris
		→ Postmenopausal pt
		→ Herpes
		
		→ Bartholin's cyst, abscess
		→ May reveal cystocele, rectocele or uterine descent / prolapse

Bimanual palpation	• Lubricate the index & middle fingers of your right hand
	• Warn pt then gently introduce fingers into vagina
	  ○ Initially palm facing left
	  ○ Slowly rotate so palm facing upwards
	• Assess vagina
	  ○ Tone
	  ○ Prolapse
	  ○ Tenderness
	  ○ Foreign bodies
	• Assess cervix
	  ○ Position
	  ○ Consistency
	  ○ Os open / closed
	  ○ Mobility (move gently between your 2 fingers)
	  ○ Excitation (tenderness)
	• Palpate uterus
	  ○ Place left hand half way between umbilicus & pubic symphysis
	  ○ Slide vaginal fingers under cervix into posterior fornix & push up
	  ○ Palpate uterus between your 2 hands
	• Assess uterus
	  ○ Size
	  ○ Shape
	  ○ Position
	  ○ Smoothness / nodularity
	  ○ Tenderness
		→ PID, ectopic pregnancy
		
		→ Anteverted/retroverted
		→ Normally smooth, nodularity caused by fibroids / malignancy
		→ e.g. adenomyosis

FEMALE GENITALIA

Bimanual palpation – cont'd	• Assess adnexae
	  ○ Move vaginal fingers into left fornix
	  ○ Move abdominal hand into left iliac fossa & press downwards
	  ○ Push vaginal fingers upwards and laterally
	  ○ Feel for masses & tenderness
	  ○ Repeat on other side
		→ Ovarian cyst, ovarian tumour, uterine fibroid, salpingitis (tender)

Speculum	• Select correct type & size of speculum
	• Lubricate blades
	• Warn pt then insert the speculum
	  ○ Ensure blades closed
	  ○ Part labia with index finger & thumb of one hand
	  ○ Introduce the speculum with the handle pointing left or right, slowly and carefully, at a downward angle
	  ○ Ensure labia & pubic hair are not caught
	  ○ Continue until flush with the perineum
	  ○ Rotate speculum 90° so handle pointing upwards
	• Locate the cervix
	  ○ Open the blades gradually until the cervix is seen
	  ○ Screw bolt down to keep speculum open
	• Inspect the cervix
	  ○ External os (morphology, open / closed)
	  ○ Erosions
	  ○ Polyps
	  ○ Growths
	  ○ Ulcers
	  ○ Discharge
	• Cervical smear test (if relevant & consented)
	  ○ Insert cytobrush through external os into endocervical canal
	  ○ Rotate through 360° 5 times
	  ○ Remove cytobrush, avoid touching speculum
	  ○ Drop cytobrush head into sample medium / rinse cytobrush in sample medium
	• Inspect vagina
	  ○ Unscrew bolt on speculum & partially close blades
	  ○ Rotate 90° (back to original insertion orientation)
	  ○ Slowly remove speculum, inspecting vaginal walls as you do
	  ○ Immediately dispose of speculum & gloves
		→ Usually use a Cusco bivalve speculum
		→ Water-based lubricant gel or water if avoiding gel (can affect some tests)
		
		→ If prolapsed vaginal walls prevent you from visualising cervix, sheath speculum with condom or finger glove with the end cut off
		
		→ Screening for cervical dyskaryosis (be familiar with your national screening programme)
		→ Method depends on sampling system being used; check expiry date
		→ Ensure vaginal walls not caught between blades

Conclusion	• Wash / gel hands, thank pt & allow to re-dress • Complete cytology paperwork if smear taken • Test vaginal pH (particularly if discharge) • Investigations: colposcopy, pelvic / transvaginal USS, vaginal swab	→ Reason for smear, LMP, OCP / HRT use → [↻]

FEMALE GENITALIA

ΔΔ Vaginal discharge

- Non-infective
  - ○ Physiological (women of reproductive age)
  - ○ Postmenopausal atrophic change
  - ○ Cervical polyps
  - ○ Cervical / uterine / ovarian malignancy
  - ○ Foreign body (e.g. retained tampon)
  - ○ Vulval dermatitis
  - ○ Fistula
- Non-sexually transmitted infection
  - ○ Bacterial vaginosis
  - ○ Thrush (Candida albicans)
- Sexually transmitted infection
  - ○ Trichomonas vaginalis
  - ○ Chlamydia trachomatis
  - ○ Neisseria gonorrhoeae

Bartholin's glands

- 2 pea-sized glands located posterior to the vaginal opening (introitus), either side of the midline
- Secrete mucous to lubricate the vagina
- Bartholin's cyst can develop if duct becomes obstructed
- Bartholin's abscess can develop if cyst become infected

NOTES

Differentiating between some infective causes of vaginal discharge

	Bacterial vaginosis	Candida albicans	Trichomonas vaginalis
Discharge	Thin white / grey	White curd-like	Frothy yellow
Odour	Fishy	Non-offensive	Offensive
Itch	Absent / minimal	Present	Present
Other symptoms		Pain Dysuria Dyspareunia	Lower abdo pain Dysuria
Possible findings on examination		Vulval erythema Oedema Fissures	Vulval inflammation Strawberry cervix
Vaginal pH	>4.5	<4.5 (normal)	>4.5

FEMALE GENITALIA NOTES

Cervical cancer

- **Risk factors**
  - Human papilloma virus infection – particularly types 16 & 18 (all girls aged 12–13 are now offered HPV vaccination in the UK)
  - Smoking
  - Immunosuppresion (HIV+, post-transplant)
  - Young age of first coitus
  - High number of sexual partners
  - Partners of promiscuous males
  - Young age of first pregnancy
  - High parity
  - Low socioeconomic class
  - Long-term OCP use
- **Symptoms**
  - Often asymptomatic – many cases detected by screening
  - Abnormal PV bleeding (postcoital, postmenopausal, intermenstrual)
  - Blood-stained vaginal discharge
  - Pelvic pain may indicate advanced disease extending beyond the cervix
- **Pathology**
  - 70–80% squamous cell carcinoma
  - 10–15% adenocarcinoma
  - Remainder melanoma, sarcoma, lymphoma
- **Management** – depending on stage of disease
  - Surgery (many options including cryotherapy, LLETZ, hysterectomy)
  - Radiotherapy often used
  - Chemotherapy in advanced / recurrent disease or where radiotherapy ineffective

BREAST EXAMINATION

	Action / Examine for	ΔΔ / Potential findings / Extra information
Introduction	<ul><li>Wash / gel hands</li><li>Introduce yourself, confirm pt, explain examination & gain consent</li><li>Ensure a chaperone is present</li><li>Expose & position pt (top and bra off, sitting on side of bed)</li><li>*"Have you noticed any breast lumps? Where is the area of concern?"*</li></ul>	
Inspection	<ul><li>Obvious lump</li><li>Skin changes</li><li>Scars from previous surgery<ul><li>Breasts</li><li>Axillae</li></ul></li><li>Compare breasts<ul><li>Hands resting by side</li><li>Hands pushing down on bed</li><li>Hands pushing in on hips</li><li>Slowly raise straight arms up above head</li></ul></li><li>Nipples<ul><li>Inversion</li><li>Discharge</li><li>Paget's disease of the nipple</li></ul></li></ul>	→ Dimpling, peau d'orange → Mastectomy, lumpectomy → Axillary node clearance → May reveal dimpling [↔] → Advanced malignant disease, normal variant → Note colour, blood-staining → Intraductal carcinoma
Palpation	<ul><li>Position pt lying flat with hand behind head on side being examined</li><li>*"Let me know if I cause you any discomfort"*</li><li>Assess each breast in turn – 'normal' one first<ul><li>Use pads of 3 middle fingers</li><li>Move systematically to ensure entire breast examined</li><li>Imagine clock face on breast, nipple at the centre – work from outside towards nipple at each point of the clock face</li><li>Palpate axillary tail</li><li>Palpate nipple & underlying tissue</li><li>If a lump is identified anywhere, assess as you would any other lump</li></ul></li><li>If pt reports nipple discharge, you can ask them to try to express some</li><li>Palpate axillary lymph nodes</li><li>Palpate lymph nodes of the head and neck</li></ul>	→ Watch pt's face for evidence of discomfort → [p94] → [p137]
Conclusion	<ul><li>Wash / gel hands, thank pt & allow them to re-dress</li><li>If not done: *"I would like to examine the other breast"*</li><li>If lump identified: *"I would go on to complete triple assessment of the breast lump by arranging imaging and fine needle aspiration"*</li><li>If malignancy suspected: *"I would like to perform a full systematic examination to look for evidence of metastatic disease"*</li></ul>	→ [↔] → Do not mention malignancy / metastasis within earshot of pt if they have not been counselled about a possible cancer diagnosis

MALE GENITALIA

	Action / Examine for	ΔΔ / Potential findings / Extra information
Introduction	• Wash / gel hands, put on non-sterile gloves • Introduce yourself, confirm pt, explain examination & gain consent • Ensure a chaperone is present • Expose & position pt (underwear removed, lying flat with 1 pillow) • *"Have you noticed any lumps in your testes? Have you had any pain in your testes? Could you point to the area of concern?"*	

Inspection	• Testes
	   ○ Enlargement / obvious mass
	   ○ Skin changes
	• Penis, groins & thighs
	   ○ Rash / infestation → Tinea, pubic lice (a highly unlikely and extremely harsh OSCE case!)
	• Ask pt to retract foreskin & inspect glans / prepuce
	   ○ Rashes
	   ○ Discharge	

Palpation	• Examine each testis in turn – 'normal' one first
	• Palpate testis with both hands between thumb and index finger
	   ○ Swelling / irregularity → Hard / soft / fluctuant / 'bag of worms' (varicocoele)
	   ○ Tenderness → Infection, testicular torsion
	• Identify spermatic cord and epididymis
	• Palpate rest of scrotum
	• If swelling identified
	   ○ Attempt to get above it → If possible excludes inguinal hernia
	   ○ Assess groins for swelling → Hernia
	         [↻]
	   ○ Identify if attached / separate to testis → Hydrocoele, epididymal cyst
	   ○ Transilluminate with torch
	   • Examine with pt standing → Varicocoele more obvious	

Conclusion	• Wash / gel hands, thank pt & allow to re-dress • If malignancy suspected: *" I would like to perform a full systemic examination to look for evidence of metastatic disease"* → Do not mention malignancy / metastasis within earshot of pt if they have not been counselled about a possible cancer diagnosis • Investigations: USS, aspiration, bloods including HCG / αFP → [↻]	

ΔΔ Breast lump
- Malignant (invasive ductal carcinoma most common)
- Benign
  - ○ Fibroadenoma
  - ○ Breast cyst (may be painful)
  - ○ Abscess (painful, hot & swollen breast)

Breast dimpling
- Does not necessarily imply invasion of cancer into underlying musculature
- Intra-mammary tumour can pull on a 'ligament of Astley Cooper', causing dimpling of the skin
- The action of raising the hands above the head tends to accentuate this

Breast cancer Rx
- Surgery
  - ○ Breast conserving
    - Lumpectomy
    - Wide local excision (if <4 cm diameter tumour)
  - ○ Mastectomy
    - Partial
    - Total
    - Radical (underlying musculature removed)
  - ○ Axillary lymph nodes
    - Sentinel node biopsy if clinically / USS node –ve
    - Axillary clearance if clinically / USS / sentinel biopsy +ve
  - ○ Breast reconstruction
    - Sometimes performed at same time as mastectomy or at a later date
- Chemotherapy
  - ○ Neo-adjuvant (pre-operative) chemotherapy may be used to shrink tumour prior to surgery
  - ○ Adjuvant (post-operative) chemotherapy following some surgery (depends on multiple factors including tumour size, grade, node & receptor status)
- Radiotherapy
  - ○ Neo-adjuvant radiotherapy not used
  - ○ Adjuvant radiotherapy following most breast-conserving surgery
  - ○ Adjuvant radiotherapy following some mastectomies (depends on multiple factors as above)
- Hormonal therapy
  - ○ Use depends on hormone receptor status of tumour
  - ○ Neo-adjuvant and adjuvant therapy can be used
  - ○ Examples: tamoxifen, anastrozole, letrozole, trastuzumab (Herceptin)

Triple assessment of a breast lump
1. Clinical examination
2. Imaging (USS / mammography)
3. Fine needle aspiration

NOTES

BREAST EXAMINATION NOTES

ΔΔ Painless scrotal swelling (excludes inguinoscrotal hernia):

	Tumour	Hydrocoele	Epididymal cyst	Varicocoele
Characteristics	Firm mass	Soft & smooth (may be large)	Soft & smooth	'Bag of worms'
Relationship to testis	Continuous	Continuous	Separate	Separate
Transillumination	–	✓✓	✓	–
Other information	Seminoma or teratoma	May be due to underlying tumour Rarely congenital	Also known as spermatocoele	Examine pt standing (may disappear when supine) More common on left* ↑incidence of infertility Rarely due to renal Ca*

ΔΔ Painful scrotal swelling
- Testicular torsion
- Torsion of testicular appendage
- Epididymo-orchitis
- Scrotal abscess
- Traumatic scrotal haematoma

Investigation of scrotal swelling
- USS
- Aspiration of fluid (not done if underlying malignancy suspected as this can disseminate malignant cells)
- Tumour markers if malignancy suspected
  - ○ αFP
  - ○ βHCG

*Varicocoele more common on left side
- Right spermatic vein drains into IVC
  - ○ Short, direct course
  - ○ Lower incidence of valvular pathology
- Left spermatic vein drains into left renal vein
  - ○ Long, tortuous course
  - ○ Valves often absent or incompetent
  - ○ Rarely, obstructed by renal Ca – new diagnosis of left varicocoele requires an abdominal USS to exclude

Testicular tumours
- Rare
- Lymphatic spread to lungs and liver
- Rx orchidectomy + chemotherapy or radiotherapy
- Seminoma (60%) – Lance Armstrong
  - ○ Age 30–40
  - ○ Highly radiosensitive
  - ○ 95% 5-year survival
- Teratoma (40%)
  - ○ Age 20–30
  - ○ Raised αFP in most
  - ○ Raised β-HCG in many
  - ○ Chemotherapy used
  - ○ 75% 5-year survival – *"terrible teratoma of the twenties"*

NOTES

DIGITAL RECTAL EXAMINATION

	Action / Examine for	ΔΔ / Potential findings / Extra information
Introduction	• Wash / gel hands, put on non-sterile gloves & apron • Introduce yourself, confirm pt, explain examination & gain consent • In particular, explain ○ The examination may be uncomfortable, but shouldn't be painful ○ There may be a feeling of rectal fullness and the need to pass stool • Ensure a chaperone is present • Expose & position pt (bare between hips & knees, left lateral position, knees pulled right up towards chin, buttocks at the edge of the examination couch)	→ Allow pt time & privacy to position themselves, and give them a blanket to cover up with before you come into the room / cubicle
Inspection	• *"First I'm going to have a look down below"* • Gently part the buttocks to expose the anus and natal cleft • Ensure good lighting & inspect carefully ○ Skin integrity & condition ○ Rash ○ Skin tags ○ Pilonidal sinus ○ Fissures & fistulae ○ Swellings protruding from anus	→ Excoriation suggests possible sphincter dysfunction & stool leakage → STI → May be a manifestation of IBD, fissure usually posterior in midline → Haemorrhoids (check if thrombosed), polyp / tumour, rectal prolapse
Palpation	• Lubricate your right index finger • Insert your finger into the rectum ○ *"I'm just about to start the internal examination now. Try to relax."* ○ Press the finger against the posterior anal margin ○ Slip the finger into the anal canal, directing the finger-tip posteriorly • Note whether the rectum is empty or loaded with faeces • Assess anal tone ○ *"Can you try to squeeze my finger?"* • Examine rectal walls ○ From the posterior starting position, slowly sweep your finger around the rectal walls, both anticlockwise and clockwise, to the anterior position ○ Ensure all 360° checked ○ To achieve this it is often necessary to move your entire upper body (e.g. turning away from the patient when sweeping anticlockwise) ○ Note the size & location of any abnormality	→ Water-based lubricant gel → Poor tone suggests neurological pathology → Use points of clock face with 12 o'clock anterior

Palpation – cont'd

- With finger in anterior position, palpate anterior structures
  - ○ ♂ Prostate
    - ■ Size → Normally ~3.5 cm (walnut size), protruding ~1 cm into rectal lumen
    - ■ Sulcus between left / right lobes → May be lost in prostatic enlargement
    - ■ Consistency → Normally rubbery & firm with no nodularity
  - ○ ♀ Possibly cervix +/– uterus (if retroverted)
- Remove finger and examine fingertip of glove
  - ○ Fresh red blood → Lower GI tract bleeding
  - ○ Melaena (black & tarry substance) → Altered blood from upper GI bleeding
  - ○ Stool
  - ○ Mucous → IBD
- Clean any lubricant / stool from around anus with a tissue
- Immediately dispose of your gloves

Conclusion

- Wash hands, thank pt & allow to re-dress
- If malignancy suspected: *"I would like to perform a full systematic examination to look for evidence of metastatic disease"* → Do not mention malignancy / metastasis within earshot of patient if they have not been counselled about a possible cancer diagnosis
- Investigations: FBC & haematinics (if evidence of GI bleeding), faecal occult blood test, sigmoidoscopy / colonoscopy, CT abdomen / pelvis

DIGITAL RECTAL EXAMINATION

Indications for digital rectal examination
- Prostatic assessment (particularly if symptoms of urinary outflow obstruction)
- Rectal bleeding
- Altered bowel habit
- Treatment-resistant constipation
- Urinary or faecal incontinence
- To check anal tone
  - Possible spinal cord pathology (traumatic or atraumatic)
  - Possible cauda equina syndrome

Causes of +ve faecal occult blood test
- Peptic ulcer
- IBD
- Polyps
- Carcinoma
- Angiodysplasia
- Swallowed blood (nose bleed, oral / dental bleeding)

Risk factors for colorectal cancer
- Personal history of colorectal cancer or polyps
- Family history of colorectal cancer or polyps
- Increasing age
- IBD
- Polyposis syndromes
- Hereditary non-polyposis colon cancer
- Female hormonal factors
  - Nulliparity
  - Late age at 1st pregnancy
  - Early menopause
- Diet
  - Rich in meat/fat
  - Poor in fibre
- Sedentary lifestyle
- Obesity
- Smoking
- High alcohol intake
- Diabetes mellitus
- Previous irradiation / asbestos exposure
- History of small bowel / endometrial / breast / ovarian cancer

DIGITAL RECTAL EXAMINATION NOTES

Surgery for colorectal carcinoma
- Right hemicolectomy: caecal, ascending proximal transverse colon tumours
- Left hemicolectomy: distal transverse & descending colon tumours
- Sigmoid colectomy: sigmoid colon tumours
- Anterior resection: low sigmoid or high rectal tumours
- Abdomino-perineal (AP) resection: low rectal tumours

NOTES

PREGNANT ABDOMEN

	Action / Examine for	ΔΔ / Potential findings / Extra information
Introduction	• Wash / gel hands • Introduce yourself, confirm pt, explain examination & gain consent • Expose pt (xiphisternum to pubic symphysis) • Position pt (semi-recumbent) • *"Do you have any pain in your tummy?"* • *"How many weeks pregnant are you?"*	→ Consider chaperone → Lying flat can obstruct IVC & cause symptomatic hypotension
The abdomen		

Inspection	• Abdominal distension
	• Fetal movements
	• Scars
	   ○ Pfannenstiel (transverse suprapubic)
	   ○ Laparotomy
	   ○ Laparoscopic
	• Cutaneous signs of pregnancy
	   ○ Linea nigra
	   ○ Striae gravidarum
	   ○ Striae albicans
	   ○ Umbilical inversion
	   ○ Dilated superficial veins
		→ The 6 Fs: Fat, Fluid, Flatus, Faeces, Fetus, Fecking big mass
		→ Usually present from about 24 wks
		→ [p16]
		→ Caesarean section
		→ Ruptured ectopic, ovarian mass removal
		→ Various gynaecological procedures
		
		→ Dark line down central abdomen from xiphisternum to pubis
		→ Purple striae (no clinical significance)
		→ Silvery-white striae (previous parity)
		→ Increased intra-abdominal pressure
		→ Collateral flow due to pressure on IVC from gravid uterus

Palpation	• Fundal height
	   ○ *"I'm going to feel for the top of your womb"*
	   ○ Use left hand, start at xiphisternum
	   ○ Work down until fundus located
	   ○ Place end of tape measure here
	   ○ Measure to pubic symphysis *with measurements facing downwards*
	   ○ Pinch tape measure at pubic symphysis & turn over to obtain measurement
	• Fetal lie (and number of fetuses)
	   ○ *"I'm now going to feel for your baby"*
	   ○ Watch pt's face throughout
	   ○ One hand each side of uterus
	   ○ Apply gentle pressure with left hand
	   ○ With right hand feel for firm, curved fetal back or lumpy fetal limbs
	   ○ Apply pressure with right hand & feel with left as above
		→ Uterus palpable from 12 wks, reaches umbilicus at 20 wks
		
		→ Avoids bias
		→ Fundal height in cm +/- 3 = weeks' gestation (after 20 wks)
		
		→ Relationship of longitudinal axes of fetus and uterus
		
		→ To ensure you do not cause any pain
		
		→ Stabilises fetus
		
		→ Lie can be longitudinal, oblique or transverse

- Presenting part
  - *"I'm going to feel deeply for the baby; if this is painful please tell me"* → Part of fetus overlying pelvic brim
  - Continue to watch pt's face
  - One hand each side of lower uterus, just above pubic symphysis
  - Apply firm pressure with both hands
  - Decide if hard, narrow & round (head) or soft and broad (bottom) → Cephalic = presenting head, breech = presenting bottom
- Engagement of the head
  - Determine cephalic presentation (as above) → 'Engaged' = widest part of fetal head has entered pelvis
  - → Not applicable if breech
  - Approximate how many finger breadths are needed to cover head above pelvic brim
  - Describe as 'fifths (of head) palpable' → One finger breadth = 1/5; ≤3/5 palpable = engaged

Auscultation
- Consider fetal lie & palpate anterior shoulder
- Pinard stethoscope → Can be used after 24 wks' gestation
  - Place bell over anterior shoulder
  - Press firmly but gently into abdomen
  - Put ear to other end
- Doppler ultrasound
  - Smear jelly on probe → Auscultate for 1 min (normal 120–140 bpm)
  - Place probe over anterior shoulder → Can be used after 18 wks' gestation
  - Adjust angle until clear heartbeat heard → Listen for 1 min (normal 120–140 bpm)

Legs
- Peripheral oedema → Can be physiological or occur with pre-eclampsia [⇨]

Conclusion
- Wash / gel hands, thank pt & allow them to re-dress
- *"I would like to perform a full cardio-respiratory examination and check the blood pressure"* → HTN may pre-date pregnancy (i.e. essential HTN) or be pregnancy-induced
- Investigations
  - Urinalysis → Proteinuria (e.g. pre-eclampsia), glycosuria (gestational DM)
  - USS
  - Cardiotocograph if any concern regarding fetal well-being (abnormal fetal heart rate, reduced fetal movements, etc.)

PREGNANT ABDOMEN

Pre-eclampsia = Pregnancy-induced hypertension + proteinuria (>0.3 g in 24 hours) +/– oedema

ΔΔ Large fundal height
- Macrosomia
- Multiple pregnancy
- Polyhydramnios

Intrauterine growth restriction
- Maternal causes
  ○ Increasing maternal age
  ○ Smoking
  ○ Alcohol
  ○ Infections (CMV, toxo, rubella, syphilis)
  ○ Diabetes mellitus (including gestational)
  ○ Renal disease
  ○ Hypertension
  ○ Thrombophilia
  ○ Drugs (warfarin, phenytoin, steroids)
- Placental causes
  ○ Pre-eclampsia
  ○ Placental abruption
- Fetal causes
  ○ Chromosomal abnormalities
  ○ Anencephaly
  ○ Multiple pregnancy

ΔΔ Small fundal height
- Fetal descent into pelvis before delivery
- Intrauterine growth retardation
- Oligohydramnios

Risk factors for breech presentation
- High maternal parity (lax uterus)
- Uterine anomaly
- Placenta praevia
- Pelvic bony abnormality
- Smoking
- Diabetes
- Fetal malformation (e.g. hydrocephalus)
- Multiple pregnancy
- Poly- or oligohydramnios
- Low birth weight (preterm or IUGR)
- Previous breech delivery

NOTES

PREGNANT ABDOMEN NOTES

Physiological changes in pregnancy
- Cardiovascular
  - Cardiac output increases 30–50% (both heart rate and stroke volume increase)
  - Reduced systemic vascular resistance due to progesterone and response to placental invasion (may cause postural hypotension)
  - BP falls during mid-pregnancy and returns to normal by week 36
  - Impaired venous return from the IVC due to pressure from the gravid uterus in late pregnancy
  - RAAS activation, salt & water retention, peripheral oedema
- Respiratory
  - Increased tidal volume
  - Compensated respiratory alkalosis (lower maternal $PaCO_2$ facilitates placental gas transfer)
- Gastrointestinal
  - Increased appetite
  - Lower oesophageal sphincter relaxation due to progesterone (predisposes to reflux)
  - Reduced GI tract motility & increased transit time (constipation common)
  - Gallbladder dilatation & incomplete emptying (predisposes to gallstone formation)
- Urinary
  - Increased renal blood flow & GFR
  - Ureteric & bladder relaxation due to progesterone (increases risk of UTI)
- Endocrine
  - Increasing progesterone & oestrogen
  - Suppressed FSH & LH
  - Increased ACTH and cortisol
  - Increased prolactin
  - Increased T4 & T3 but also increased thyroxine-binding globulin
  - Reduced peripheral insulin sensitivity (predisposes to gestational diabetes)
- Haematological
  - Increased plasma volume & dilutional anaemia
  - Slightly raised white cell count
  - Reduced serum iron, increased transferrin & TIBC
  - Increased clotting factors (VII, VIII, IX, X) & reduced fibrinolytic activity ($\uparrow$ VTE risk)
- Skin
  - Hyperpigmentation of umbilicus, nipples, abdominal midline (linea nigra) & face (chloasma)
  - Striae gravidarum
  - Palmar erythema (hyperdynamic circulation)
- Musculoskeletal
  - Increased ligament laxity (causes back pain & pubic symphysis dysfunction)
  - Exaggerated lumbar lordosis in late pregnancy

NOTES

	Action / Examine for	ΔΔ / Potential findings / Extra information

Introduction	• Wash / gel hands
	• Introduce yourself to parents, explain examination & gain consent
	• Check mother's identity & check baby's wrist bands
	• Ask mother to strip baby down to nappy & place on changing mat
	• Meanwhile ask
	  ○ *"How, when and at what gestation was the baby born?"*
	  ○ *"Any problems with mum or baby during pregnancy / labour / delivery?"*
	  ○ *"Is he / she feeding OK? Passing pee and black poo?"*
	  ○ *"Are there any congenital conditions in either parent's family?"*
	  ○ *"Do you have any particular concerns about the baby?"*
		→ Neonatal examination should be done within 72 hours of birth
		
		→ Should urinate within first 24 hours & pass meconium within 48 hours

General observation	• Skin (jaundice, cyanosis, bruising) • Tone • Sleepiness / rousability • Nature of cry • Measure weight & length • Check temperature	→ Ideally examine in bright daylight; bruising may be from birth trauma → Floppiness is abnormal (e.g. septic, CNS pathology, Down's syndrome) → Compare to centile chart → Sepsis
Head	• Inspect head size & shape • Measure head circumference • Palpate fontanelles (normal / sunken / bulging)	→ May be moulding from vaginal delivery → Refer to centile chart → Sunken suggests dehydration, bulging when not crying suggests raised ICP

Face	• Inspect general facial appearance & symmetry
	• Eyes
	  ○ Position, symmetry, size & shape
	  ○ Check for red reflex using ophthalmoscope
	• Ears
	  ○ Position, symmetry, size & shape
	  ○ Patency of external auditory meatus
	• Mouth
	  ○ Put clean little finger inside mouth & feel entire palate
	  ○ Tongue tie
		→ Normal or dysmorphic
		
		→ Down's syndrome [⇔]
		→ Normally red, absent with congenital cataracts, white with retinoblastoma
		
		→ Cleft palate, high-arched palate (Down's syndrome, Marfan's syndrome)

Upper limbs	• Inspect size, shape, symmetry, deformity & movement • Count fingers • Count palmar creases	→ Abnormal posture, e.g. Erb's palsy → Extra digits (polydactyly), fused digits (syndactyly) → Single palmar crease can be associated with Down's syndrome [⇔]
Cardiovascular	• Palpate femoral, brachial & radial pulses (rate / rhythm / volume) • Radio-radial & radio-femoral delay • Check central CRT on sternum • Palpate precordium for heart position / heaves / thrills • Auscultate heart	→ Normally 110–160 bpm; PDA causes bounding pulses → Aortic coarctation → Dextrocardia → Neonatal stethoscope; consider causes of murmur [⇔]

NEONATAL

Respiratory	• Note respiratory pattern & depth of breathing • Listen for stridor / grunting • Look for nasal flaring / intercostal indrawing • Auscultate breath sounds & count respiratory rate	→ Airway obstruction, respiratory distress → Respiratory distress → Normally 30–60 bpm
Abdomen	• Inspect for distension • Check umbilicus for hernia / infection • Palpate abdomen for organomegaly / masses	→ Common to feel liver and/or spleen in healthy neonates
Genitalia & anus	• Inspect carefully & check anus patent • Palpate testes in boy	→ Clear male/female or ambiguous; exclude hypospadias in boys → Undescended testes
Back	• Inspect skin for defects & tufts of hair • Inspect spinal symmetry & curvatures • Palpate spine	→ Meningocele / myelomeningocele / spina bifida occulta → Spina bifida occulta

Lower limbs	• Inspect size & shape, symmetry, deformity & movement
	• Count toes
	• Hips
	  ○ Barlow's test (each leg in turn)
	    ■ Baby's knees flexed, hold thighs (your thumbs medial & index / middle fingers lateral)
	    ■ Flex hip to 90°, ADduct & push leg downwards
	    ■ Click indicates hip *dislocation*
	  ○ Ortolani's test (each leg in turn)
	    ■ Same starting position as for Barlow's test
	    ■ Flex hip to 90°, slowly ABduct fully whilst applying anterior force to greater trochanter with your index / middle fingertips
	    ■ Click indicates hip *relocation*
		→ Talipes equinovarus (club foot) = inversion & high medial arch
		→ Identifies unstable hip by dislocating it (i.e. DDH [↪])
		→ I.e. apply a posterior dislocating force to the femur
		→ Identifies unstable hip that is already dislocated by relocating it (i.e. DDH)
		Ortolani = **Out**

Primitive reflexes	• Moro reflex
	  ○ Explain to parents first
	  ○ Hold baby in front of you, just above mat, sitting on your hand
	  ○ With your other hand support back, neck and head
	  ○ Suddenly drop upper body backward and downwards
	  ○ Arms should ABduct & extend then ADduct & flex (baby may then cry)
	• Grasp reflex
	  ○ Place a finger in baby's palm and he / she should grasp the finger
	• Suckling reflex
	  ○ Place a clean finger in baby's mouth, touch palate and he/she should suck the finger
		→ All of these reflexes should be present from birth
		→ Absence usually suggests CNS pathology, although unilateral absence of Moro may occur due to brachial plexus pathology
		→ Some clinicians would only perform if suspicion of CNS pathology, but it is important to know them for OSCEs

Conclusion	• Wash / gel hands, thank parents & allow to re-dress baby • Update parents with findings & whether further review / action required • Investigations: hip USS (if DDH suspected), bloods	

NEONATAL

Apgar scoring
- Quantitative assessment of neonatal condition after delivery
- 5 clinical features scored 0, 1 or 2
- Maximum score 10 (however, normal babies achieve maximum of 9 as have blue extremities)
- Useful for assessing neonate's progress or deterioration
- Checked at 1 then 5 minutes after delivery (additional checks every 5 minutes until score >6)
- Infants with Apgar <7 at 5 minutes have increased mortality & severe neurological morbidity

Score	0	1	2
Appearance (colour)	Blue, pale	Body pink, extremities blue	Completely pink
Pulse rate	Absent	<100 bpm	>100 bpm
Grimace (reflex irritability – response to plantar stimulation)	Absent	Grimace	Cry
Activity (muscle tone)	Limp	Some flexion of extremities	Active motion
Respiratory effort	Absent	Slow or irregular breaths	Good strong cry & adequate respiratory effort

Developmental dysplasia of the hip (DDH)
- Affects 1–3% of neonates
- Left hip dislocated more often than right
- 20% bilateral
- Risk factors
  - Girls (80% of cases)
  - First-born
  - Breech delivery (vaginal or caesarean section)
  - Oligohydramnios (restricted movement *in utero*)
  - Multiple pregnancy
  - Prematurity
  - Neuromuscular disorder
  - Family history of DDH
- Indications for hip USS
  - Family history of DDH or possible DDH (hip problems in early life)
  - Fetus that was breech at any point after 36 weeks gestation
  - Fetus that was breech at delivery if delivery before 36 weeks gestation
  - Suspicion of DDH on clinical testing
- Management
  - Most unstable hips stabilise spontaneously by 2–6 weeks of age
  - Harness/splint used to maintain hip reduction as soon as diagnosis confirmed
  - Surgery
    - No response to early harness / splint
    - Late diagnosis and not suitable for harness / splint

NOTES

NEONATAL NOTES

Down's syndrome

- Genetics
  - 95% trisomy 21 (chromosome count 47)
  - 5% translocation (chromosome count 46)
  - Mosaicism can occur
- Facial features
  - Brachycephaly (wide, flat head)
  - Short neck
  - Epicanthic folds on medial aspect of eyes
  - Downward slant to eyes medially
  - Small ears, which may be low-set
  - Flat nasal bridge
  - Mouth hanging open
  - Large, often protruding tongue
  - Narrow high arched palate
  - Transverse tongue fissures
- Other possible features in neonate
  - Hypotonia
  - Short fingers (particularly short / absent middle phalanx of little finger)
  - Clinodactyly (curved digits)
  - Single palmar crease
  - Wide space between 1st & 2nd toes
  - Congenital heart lesions
- Features developing later in life
  - Learning difficulties
  - Cataracts
  - Associated disorders
    - Hypothyroidism
    - Visual impairment
    - Hearing impairment
    - Leukaemia
    - Obstructive sleep apnoea

ΔΔ Neonatal murmur

- PDA (normally closes by 48 hours post-delivery)
- Other structural heart disease
- Innocent murmur (produced by normal blood flow through heart)

Edward's syndrome

- Genetics
  - Trisomy 18 (47 chromosomes)
  - Mosaicism can occur
  - Affects females more than males
- Facial features
  - Microcephaly with prominent occiput
  - Low-set dysplastic ears
  - Crowded face
  - Micrognathia
  - Small eyes
- Other features in neonate
  - Flexed & overlapping fingers
  - Rockerbottom feet
  - Cryptorchidism (testes not in scrotum)
  - Low birth weight
  - Congenital heart lesions (especially VSD)
  - Apnoeic episodes

Neonatal blood screening ('heel prick' test)

- Usually taken on day 5 post-delivery
- Conditions tested for
  - Sickle cell disease
  - Cystic fibrosis
  - Congenital hypothyroidism
  - Phenylketonuria (PKU)
  - Medium-chain acyl-coenzyme A dehydrogenase deficiency (MCADD)
  - Maple syrup urine disease (MSUD)
  - Isovaleric acidaemia (IVA)
  - Glutaric aciduria type 1 (GA1)
  - Homocystinuria (HCU)

NOTES

- ABCDE approach. Treat problems as you identify them; don't move on from life-threatening problems until they are resolved (or at least improving following intervention).
- If clinical picture changes or you complete an intervention, |REASSESS| (e.g. after a fluid challenge). Go back to Airway if necessary.
- At all times consider whether you need **help**. How unwell is the patient? Do you need someone with more experience or specific skills? Do you simply need more hands? If so, state clearly that you would call for help, who you would call and why.

	Action / Examine for	ΔΔ / Potential findings / Extra information
Introduction	• Wash / gel hands, put on gloves / apron if necessary • Introduce yourself, confirm, explain examination & gain consent • Obtain quick background history from whoever has been with pt • Ask nurse: *"Put on a sats probe, attach 3-lead ECG & check BP please"*	→ May not be possible if pt drowsy / confused → Nursing staff, paramedic, family, carer → If automatic BP you could set to cycle every 2 mins at first

Assessment	• Conscious patient: *"Hello, how are you?"*
	  ○ Exclude signs of obstruction
	    ■ *Look* for visible swelling of lips / tongue
	    ■ *Listen* for stridor / snoring
	• Unconscious patient: confirm respiratory effort (chest moving)
	  ○ Exclude signs of obstruction
	    ■ *Look* for paradoxical 'see-saw' chest / abdominal movement
	    ■ *Look* for vomit / foreign body in the mouth & remove
	    ■ *Listen* for stridor / snoring / gurgling
		→ If patient answers, they probably have a clear airway, are definitely breathing and are perfusing their brain
		→ E.g. anaphylaxis
		→ If absent, call resus team, check pulse & follow ALS / BLS algorithm
		→ Suction vomit, remove chunks / foreign body with Magill forceps
		→ However, in complete airway obstruction there will be *no noise*

Consider interventions	• Apply oxygen (e.g. 15 l/min via a non-rebreather mask) • Open airway if unresponsive & airway obstructed • Call anaesthetist if stridor or ongoing airway manoeuvres required	→ [↻] → Head tilt & chin lift, jaw thrust, consider adjuncts (e.g. Guedel airway) → May require advanced airway management (e.g. endotracheal intubation)

A AIRWAY

- If patient is conscious, talking, with an uncompromised airway, you could take a brief history (e.g. SAMPLE [↻]) which will help guide further assessment
- If this takes longer than a minute or two to get, don't delay moving on to BCDE – you can continue to build up the history as you assess

Assessment	• Respiratory rate • Oxygen saturations • Check trachea is central • Inspect chest wall for deformity or subcutaneous emphysema • Look for accessory muscle use • Assess adequacy and symmetry of chest expansion • Percuss & auscultate chest	→ ↑ respiratory rate is a useful indicator of how unwell the patient is → Deviated towards collapse / pneumonectomy, away from tension / effusion → Subcutaneous emphysema = pneumothorax until proven otherwise → May only be able to percuss / auscultate from anterior if pt cannot sit up
Investigations	• ABG • CXR	→ Useful in almost any critically ill patient
Consider interventions	• Nebulisers for wheeze • Needle decompression of tension pneumothorax	→ Asthma / COPD or anaphylaxis (consider other signs & context) → Do *not* wait for CXR if pt hypoxic or hypotensive

B BREATHING

CRITICALLY ILL PATIENT

CRITICALLY ILL PATIENT

C CIRCULATION

Assessment
- Temperature of peripheries & CRT → Check both hands & feet
- Radial pulse (rate, rhythm, volume) → Use more proximal pulses if difficult to palpate
- Blood pressure → Compare to pt's normal BP if known
- JVP → Very high in severe asthma, tension pneumothorax, tamponade
- Auscultate heart sounds → Only necessary if specific concerns (e.g. ?LVF, ?acute MR post-MI)

Investigations
- Bloods → Can usually be taken when IV access is obtained [⟳]
- 12-lead ECG → Perform if chest pain, tachy-/bradycardia, irregular pulse, possible high K+

Consider interventions
- Obtain IV access (consider IO if IV difficult) → ≥16G (grey) if shock / bleeding, x 2 if major haemorrhage
- If hypovolaemic, administer a fluid challenge then REASSESS → [⟳] Consider major haemorrhage protocol if bleeding & shocked
- Catheter & hourly urine output

D DISABILITY

Assessment
- Conscious level (AVPU or GCS) → AVPU is simple & quick, GCS takes practice to perform rapidly
- Pupils (size, symmetry, reactivity to light)
- Neurological examination of limbs if indicated / possible → Suspected neurological pathology (e.g. stroke, intracranial bleed)

Investigations
- Blood glucose (bedside measurement) → Administer glucose if <4 mmol/l ('four's the floor')

Consider interventions
- Glucose → Oral if conscious & alert, otherwise IV
- Naloxone / flumazenil → Opioid / benzodiazepine toxicity

E EXPOSURE

Assessment
- Measure core temperature → Level of detail will depend on how concerned you are about pathology
- Expose & examine abdomen / limbs / surgical wounds / drains → Rash, jaundice, trauma, bruising
- Expose & examine skin

Investigations
- Cultures (blood +/- urine, sputum, stool, wound swab, etc.) → If pyrexial or possible sepsis; take *before* giving antibiotics unless delay

Consider interventions
- Antibiotics → Consult local guidelines
- Analgesia → If severe pain give IV opioid (e.g. morphine) titrated to effect

Obtain more information
- Review charts: observation, medication, fluid balance
- Collateral history if not already known

STOP AND THINK
- What is the working diagnosis? What is in the differential diagnosis? → Speak these thoughts out loud, invite other team members to contribute
- Considering this:
  - What further investigations are needed? → e.g. CT head +/- lumbar puncture, CT abdomen / pelvis, PEFR
  - What further interventions are needed? → e.g. ACS treatment, anticonvulsants
  - Who do you need to contact? → e.g. your senior, a surgeon, an anaesthetist, critical care team
  - Where does the patient need to go? → e.g. HDU, ICU, cardiac cath lab for PCI, theatre

REASSESS

Oxygen therapy
- Patients die from hypoxia
- In general, critically ill patients should receive oxygen to maximise tissue oxygen delivery
- Oxygen can later be titrated down if the patient is stable
- 2 situations require further consideration:
  1. **COPD**: some patients rely on hypoxic drive as a stimulus to breathe because they have become desensitised to chronic hypercapnia (this includes a subgroup of COPD patients). Administration of excessive O_2 may result in hypoventilation, worsening hypercapnia and narcosis. If pt has COPD, use controlled O_2 therapy and titrate to SpO_2 88–92% (e.g. start with 28% Venturi mask). If SpO_2 falls well below this, go back to 15 l/min O_2 via a non-rebreather mask then titrate back down once oxygenation improves.
  2. **ACS**: there is some evidence that excessive O_2 can cause harm in the context of ACS. Consequently, current UK guidance is that in patients with possible cardiac chest pain supplemental O_2 should only be administered if SpO_2 <94%, aiming for SpO_2 94–98%. In COPD patients at risk of hypercapnic respiratory failure (see point 1) use controlled O_2 therapy aim for SpO_2 88–92%. [NICE 2010, CG95]

Fluid challenge
- Shock is defined as inadequate tissue perfusion
- Signs of shock include
  - Cool peripheries
  - Prolonged CRT >2 sec
  - Tachycardia
  - Confusion / reduced conscious level (cerebral hypoperfusion)
  - Oliguria / anuria (renal hypoperfusion)
  - Hypotension (*late* sign, particularly in young fit patients)
- If pt has signs of shock or hypovolaemia, give a fluid challenge over 5–10 min, for example:
  - 1000 ml of crystalloid (ideally warmed) if hypotensive
  - 500 ml of crystalloid (ideally warmed) if normotensive
  - 250 ml of crystalloid (ideally warmed) if background of cardiac disease or frail
- Which crystalloid?
  - Balanced solution if no concern about possible hyperkalaemia (e.g. Plasma-Lyte 148)
  - 0.9% NaCl if known or possible hyperkalaemia (consider patient context)
- Ways to ensure a fluid challenge can be given quickly
  - Big peripheral venous cannula, ideally ≥16G (grey) – if not then the biggest you can get in
  - Big vein
  - Big giving set (e.g. blood giving set)
  - Pressurise the fluids (squeeze manually or use a pressure bag)
- Following the fluid challenge, REASSESS and make an ongoing plan
  - If significant, sustained improvement, continue to monitor
  - If partial / unsustained / no improvement and no signs of fluid overload, repeat challenge*
  - If fluid overload (↑RR, ↓SpO_2, ↑SOB, basal creps, ↑JVP) stop fluids & seek senior advice

*If pt shocked due to haemorrhage, particularly if still actively bleeding, they likely need *blood* – request blood early and consider activating a major haemorrhage protocol if available

CRITICALLY ILL PATIENT NOTES

Sepsis six [Emerg Med J. 2011;28:507]
- 3 'tests' & 3 'treatments'
  1. Take blood cultures
  2. Measure blood lactate & Hb
  3. Catheterise & hourly urine output
  4. High flow O_2
  5. IV fluid challenges
  6. Broad spectrum antibiotics
- Start as soon as sepsis is identified in ΔΔ
- If you have performed a thorough ABCDE assessment you will achieve these anyway, but it is useful to have a check list

Selected blood tests & possible indications
- Full blood count
  ○ Any unwell patient (?anaemia, ?sepsis)
  ○ Bleeding patient (?thrombocytopaenia)
- Urea & electrolytes
  ○ Any unwell patient (?AKI)
  ○ Arrhythmia (?electrolyte disturbance)
- Liver function tests
  ○ ?hepatobiliary disease
- C-reactive protein
  ○ ?sepsis
- Lactate
  ○ ?sepsis
- Troponin
  ○ ?ACS
- Coagulation screen
  ○ ?hepatobiliary disease
  ○ Bleeding patient (?coagulopathic)
- Group & save
  ○ Small bleed now stopped
  ○ Possibly requires surgery
- Cross-match
  ○ Large bleed & hypovolaemic pt
  ○ Ongoing significant bleeding

SAMPLE history
- Symptoms
- Allergies
- Medications
- Past medical history
- Last ate / drank
- Events leading to this point

Possible OSCE scenarios
- Acute coronary syndrome
- Tachyarrhythmia
- Bradyarrhythmia
- Acute asthma exacerbation
- Acute COPD exacerbation
- Pneumothorax +/– tension
- Pulmonary embolism
- GI bleed
- Intracranial bleed
- Ischaemic stroke
- Seizure
- Post-ictal state
- Opioid overdose
- Burns
- Acute abdomen
- Hyperkalaemia
- Sepsis
  ○ Pneumonia
  ○ Urinary tract infection
  ○ Intra-abdominal source
  ○ Cellulitis / soft tissue infection
  ○ Meningoencephalitis
- Head injury*
- Other trauma +/– haemorrhage*

*Trauma resuscitation incorporates additional elements such as cervical spine control, and is beyond the scope of this book.

	Action / Examine for	ΔΔ / Potential findings / Extra information

Introduction	• Wash / gel hands
	• Confirm pt identity (wrist band)
	• Obtain background information from nursing staff / notes
	• Establish that one of the following is applicable
	  ○ 'Do Not Attempt Resuscitation' decision made
	  ○ Cardiopulmonary resuscitation attempts failed
	  ○ Life-sustaining treatment has been actively withdrawn
		→ If any uncertainty, commence CPR whilst awaiting clarification

Assessment	• Over **5 min**, repeatedly check for absence of the following
	  ○ Visible respiratory effort
	  ○ Breath sounds
	  ○ Heart sounds
	  ○ Carotid pulse
	• If no signs of cardiorespiratory activity after 5 min check
	  ○ Pupillary responses using pen torch
	  ○ Corneal reflex using wisp of cotton wool
	  ○ Response to pain using supraorbital pressure
	• Following all of the above note the time of death
		→ Time the 5 min
		
		→ Must be fixed & dilated
		→ Must be no blinking
		→ Must be no movement

Conclusion	• Wash / gel hands • Update nursing staff • Ensure next of kin informed & offer to speak with them • Notify responsible consultant & confirm details for death certificate • Complete death certificate if appropriate • Notify GP	→ Cause of death, etc. → Not if referral to coroner / procurator fiscal is required
Documentation	• Patient identifiers on top of page • Date & time • Your name & grade • Write each step of the assessment above & the result • Date & time when death confirmed • Sign, print & write your GMC number	

[Acad Med R Coll 2008, A code of practice for the diagnosis and confirmation of death]

CONFIRMING DEATH

APPENDICES

Lymph node groups

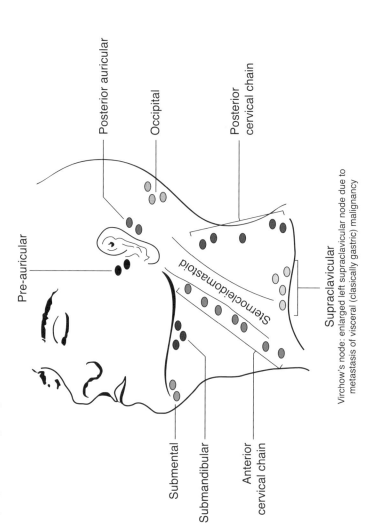

Posterior auricular

Occipital

Posterior cervical chain

Pre-auricular

Sternocleidomastoid

Supraclavicular

Submental

Submandibular

Anterior cervical chain

Virchow's node: enlarged left supraclavicular node due to metastasis of visceral (clasically gastric) malignancy

ΔΔ Lymphadenopathy

1. Localised
- Acute local infection (e.g. tonsillitis)
- Neoplastic
  - Local malignancy
  - Solitary distant metastasis

2. Generalised
- Acute generalised infection
  - EBV
  - HIV seroconversion
- Chronic infection
  - TB 'cold abscesses'
  - Syphilis
  - HIV
- Neoplastic
  - Multiple distant metastases
  - Haematological
    - lymphoma
    - CLL
- Systemic disease
  - Sarcoidosis
  - RA

Typical characteristics of lymphadenopathy

- Tender & fluctuant: Acute infection
- Non-tender & rubbery: Lymphoma / CLL
- Non-tender & hard: Metastatic

LYMPH NODES OF THE HEAD AND NECK

Examining the lymph nodes of the head and neck

Examination of the lymph nodes of the head and neck is a key component of several examinations. To begin, stand behind the pt and place both hands under their chin (over the submental nodes). Using the pads of your index, middle and ring fingers feel carefully in the sequence shown below. Examine both sides simultaneously. If you detect lymphadenopathy, assess the enlarged lymph node as you would any other lump [p94].

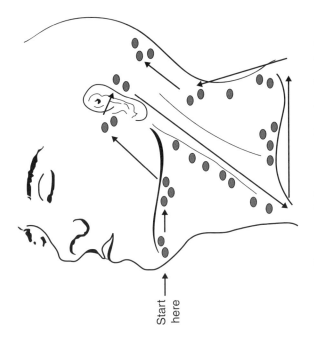

Start here

Recommended sequence of lymph node palpation

1. Submental
2. Submandibular
3. Pre-auricular
4. Posterior auricular
5. Anterior cervical chain
6. Supraclavicular
7. Posterior cervical chain
8. Occipital

LYMPH NODES OF THE HEAD AND NECK

The following clinical signs come up time and time again due to their association with various diseases of multiple systems. Their causes are essential to know well.

Features of finger clubbing
- Increased fluctuance of nailbed
- Loss of nailbed angle
- Increased longitudinal curvature of nail
- Drumsticking

ΔΔ Finger clubbing
Systems implicated: cardiovascular, respiratory, gastrointestinal, endocrine

- Cardiovascular disease
  - Cyanotic congenital heart disease
  - Infective endocarditis
  - Atrial myxoma
- Respiratory disease
  - Interstitial lung disease
  - Malignancy
    - bronchogenic carcinoma
    - mesothelioma
  - Suppurative lung disease
    - bronchiectasis *(pus in the tubes)*
    - abscess *(pus in a collection)*
    - empyema *(pus outside the lung)*
    - cystic fibrosis *(pus everywhere)*
- Gastrointestinal disease
  - IBD
  - Hepatic cirrhosis
  - GI lymphoma
  - Coeliac disease
- Other causes
  - Thyroid acropachy (Graves' disease)
  - Familial

KEY DIFFERENTIAL DIAGNOSES

ΔΔ Ankle swelling

Systems implicated: cardiovascular, respiratory, gastrointestinal, renal, endocrine, vascular

- Pitting oedema
  - Raised venous pressure
    - chronic venous insufficiency
    - right heart failure
    - volume overload (e.g. renal failure)
    - immobility
    - constrictive pericarditis
    - obesity (with associated Na^+ / H_2O retention)
    - pregnancy
  - Reduced oncotic pressure (hypoalbuminaemia)
    - nephrotic syndrome
    - cirrhosis / liver failure
    - severe malnutrition
    - protein-losing enteropathy (e.g. IBD)
    - exfoliative dermatitis
  - Drug-related
    - calcium channel blockers
    - long-term corticosteroids [p84]
    - NSAIDs

- Non-pitting oedema
  - Lymphoedema
    - primary (e.g. Milroy's disease)
    - malignancy
    - filariasis
    - radiotherapy
    - lymph node clearance
  - Hypothyroidism
  - Pre-tibial myxoedema (Graves' disease)

- Unilateral / localised swelling
  - Acute DVT
  - Post-thrombotic syndrome
  - Associated with cellulitis

KEY DIFFERENTIAL DIAGNOSES

3rd Yr OSCE

10 bays - 8min + 2 min move

3 x pt - examination

3x role play - history

1) Practical procedure

1) Case discussion

2x data interpretation /
    unprepared case discussion